Forensic Psychiatry

Guest Editors

WILLIAM BERNET, MD
BRADLEY W. FREEMAN, MD

CHILD AND ADOLESCENT PSYCHIATRIC CLINICS OF NORTH AMERICA

www.childpsych.theclinics.com

Consulting Editor
HARSH K. TRIVEDI, MD

July 2011 • Volume 20 • Number 3

SAUNDERS an imprint of ELSEVIER, Inc.

W.B. SAUNDERS COMPANY
A Division of Elsevier Inc.

Elsevier Inc. • 1600 John F. Kennedy Boulevard • Suite 1800 • Philadelphia, Pennsylvania 19103-2899

http://www.childpsych.theclinics.com

CHILD AND ADOLESCENT PSYCHIATRIC CLINICS OF NORTH AMERICA Volume 20, Number 3
July 2011 ISSN 1056–4993, ISBN-13: 978-1-4557-1024-9

Editor: Sarah E. Barth
Developmental Editor: Donald Mumford

Child and Adolescent Psychiatric Clinics of North America (ISSN 1056-4993) is published quarterly by Elsevier Inc., 360 Park Avenue South, New York, NY 10010-1710. Months of issue are January, April, July, and October. Business and Editorial Offices: 1600 John F. Kennedy Boulevard, Suite 1800, Philadelphia, PA 19103-2899. Periodicals postage paid at New York, NY and additional mailing offices. Subscription prices are $275.00 per year (US individuals), $425.00 per year (US institutions), $139.00 per year (US students), $318.00 per year (Canadian individuals), $513.00 per year (Canadian institutions), $176.00 per year (Canadian students), $378.00 per year (international individuals), $513.00 per year (international institutions), and $176.00 per year (international students). International air speed delivery is included in all Clinics subscription prices. All prices are subject to change without notice. **POSTMASTER:** Send address changes to Child and Adolescent Psychiatric Clinics of North America, Elsevier Health Sciences Division, Subscription Customer Service, 3251 Riverport Lane, Maryland Heights, MO 63043. **Customer Service: 1-800-654-2452 (U.S. and Canada); 314-447-8871 (outside U.S. and Canada). Fax: 314-447-8029. E-mail: JournalsCustomerService-usa@ elsevier.com (for print support) or journalsonlinesupport-usa@elsevier.com (for online support).**

Reprints. For copies of 100 or more of articles in this publication, please contact the Commercial Reprints Department, Elsevier Inc., 360 Park Avenue South, New York, New York 10010-1710 Tel.: (212) 633-3812; Fax: (212) 462-1935, e-mail: reprints@elsevier.com.

Child and Adolescent Psychiatric Clinics of North America is covered in *MEDLINE/PubMed (Index Medicus), ISI, SSCI, Research Alert, Social Search, Current Contents,* and *EMBASE/Excerpta Medica.*

Printed in the United States of America.

Contributors

CONSULTING EDITOR

HARSH K. TRIVEDI, MD
Associate Professor of Psychiatry, Vanderbilt University School of Medicine; and
Executive Medical Director, and Chief of Staff, Vanderbilt Psychiatric Hospital,
Nashville, Tennessee

CONSULTING EDITOR EMERITUS

ANDRÉS MARTIN, MD, MPH

FOUNDING CONSULTING EDITOR

MELVIN LEWIS, MBBS, FRCPSYCH, DCH

GUEST EDITORS

WILLIAM BERNET, MD
Professor, Department of Psychiatry, Vanderbilt University School of Medicine, Nashville,
Tennessee

BRADLEY W. FREEMAN, MD
Assistant Professor, Department of Psychiatry, Vanderbilt University School of Medicine,
Nashville, Tennessee

AUTHORS

PETER ASH, MD
Director, Psychiatry and Law Service; Chief, Division of Child and Adolescent
Psychiatry; Associate Professor, Department of Psychiatry and Behavioral Sciences,
Emory University, Atlanta, Georgia

PAUL BENSUSSAN, MD
Private Practice; National Psychiatric Expert Appointed by the *Cour de cassation*
(the French Supreme Court), Versailles, France

WILLIAM BERNET, MD
Professor, Department of Psychiatry, Vanderbilt University School of Medicine, Nashville,
Tennessee

JEFF Q. BOSTIC, MD, EdD
Director of School Psychiatry; Associate Clinical Professor; Medical Director of the Massachusetts Child Psychiatry Access Project Site at MGH, Department of Psychiatry, Massachusetts General Hospital, Harvard Medical School, Boston, Massachusetts

COLBY C. BRUNT, JD
Stoneman, Chandler and Miller, Boston, Massachusetts

JOSHUA W. BUCKHOLTZ, PhD
Department of Psychology; Vanderbilt Brain Institute, Vanderbilt University, Nashville, Tennessee; Department of Psychology, Harvard University, Cambridge, Massachusetts

DAVID L. CORWIN, MD
Professor of Pediatrics and Chief, Pediatrics' Child Protection and Family Health Division, University of Utah School of Medicine; Medical Director, Primary Children's Center for Safe and Healthy Families, Salt Lake City, Utah

DOUGLAS DARNALL, PhD
Psychologist, CEO, PsyCare, Inc, Youngstown, Ohio

R. GREGG DWYER, MD, EdD
Associate Professor, Department of Psychiatry and Behavioral Sciences; Forensic Psychiatry Program Director and Sexual Behaviors Clinic and Lab Director, Medical University of South Carolina, Charleston, South Carolina

BRADLEY W. FREEMAN, MD
Assistant Professor, Department of Psychiatry, Vanderbilt University School of Medicine, Nashville, Tennessee

BROOKS R. KEESHIN, MD
Fellow, Child Abuse Pediatrics, Mayerson Center for Safe and Healthy Families, Cincinnati Children's Hospital Medical Center, Cincinnati, Ohio

ELIZABETH J. LETOURNEAU, PhD
Associate Professor, Department of Psychiatry and Behavioral Sciences, Family Services Research Center, Medical University of South Carolina, Charleston, South Carolina

STEPHEN A. MONTGOMERY, MD
Assistant Professor, Department of Psychiatry, Vanderbilt University School of Medicine, Nashville, Tennessee

PAUL J. O'LEARY, MD
Fellow in Forensic Psychiatry, Psychiatry and Law Service, Department of Psychiatry and Behavioral Sciences, Emory University, Atlanta, Georgia

CHARLES SCOTT, MD
Professor of Clinical Psychiatry and Chief, Division of Psychiatry and the Law, Department of Psychiatry and Behavioral Sciences, University of California, Davis Medical Center, Sacramento, California

DAVID M. SIEGEL, JD
Professor of Law, New England Law, Boston; Co-Director, Center for Law and Social Responsibility, Boston, Massachusetts

DAVID F. STREET, MD
Assistant Professor, Department of Psychiatry, Vanderbilt University School of Medicine, Nashville, Tennessee

MICHAEL T. TREADWAY, MA
Department of Psychology, Vanderbilt University, Nashville, Tennessee

JAMES S. WALKER, PhD
Adjunct Assistant Professor, Department of Psychology, Vanderbilt University; Private Practice of Neuropsychology; Neuropsychology Consultants, PLLC, Nashville, Tennessee

Contents

Specialized interventions for juveniles who have committed sex offenses have been widely available for 25 years. These interventions initially were based largely on adult sex offender interventions, with little consideration of developmental and other differences that distinguish juveniles from adult offenders. More recently, interventions have been developed that address youth-specific factors associated with problem sexual behaviors and that include a stronger family focus. This article reviews the history of intervention approaches, summarizes specialized evaluation methods and addresses the assessment of juvenile recidivism risk.

The US Supreme Court has set 2 key constitutionally based limits to punishment of juveniles; a bar on the imposition of the death penalty for crimes committed by juveniles and of life imprisonment without possibility of parole for juveniles who commit nonhomicide offenses. Both decisions held that these penalties were disproportionate given juveniles' distinctive characteristics. The Court's adoption of a developmental model of culpability may produce future challenges to lengthy juvenile sentences, broad provisions allowing transfer of juveniles for trial as adults, and even possibly to younger juveniles'competence to stand trial.

Bullying is an abuse of power and control that can cause significant harm to individuals. School systems have the difficult task of trying to police this behavior to maintain a safe learning environment for their students. Although there may be an identified bully, the ramifications of the behavior affect the system as a whole. Bullies, targeted victims, and bystanders play an integral role in ameliorating this problem. A change of culture within the school system is often the best, yet often the most difficult, intervention. In addition, cyberbullying has become a powerful avenue for bullying, resulting in significant morbidity within schools.

Contact refusal is a common phenomenon that can occur during the course of, or after, divorce, which affects the relationship between a child and the parent. This article defines the concept of contact refusal and discusses the importance of its recognition. The concept is further narrowed to focus on the child as the one refusing contact, not the parent, which can happen as well. Various types of contact refusals are illustrated in the article through clinical vignettes, and an approach to categorizing the various types of contact refusal is presented.

Parental alienation occurs in divorces when one parent indoctrinates the child to dislike, fear, and avoid contact with the other parent. Mental health professionals who treat children and adolescents are likely to encounter victims of parental alienation in clinical practice, and it is important to identify and treat these youngsters earlier, when the condition is mild, rather than later, when the parental alienation is almost intractable. This article presents an overview of the treatment of parental alienation, which is called reunification therapy. All the parties involved in the case have a role in the prevention and treatment of parental alienation.

Forensic mental health professionals are frequently asked to evaluate the parenting skills of divorcing parents because the court seeks help in determining the custody, visitation, and parenting time arrangements for the children. When one of the parents is impaired, the court wants to know the way to help the children have a good relationship with that parent and keep the children safe. There is little empirical research to answer such questions. In this article, the authors describe their methodology for providing useful clinical information to the court to help guide their decisions regarding visitation with impaired parents.

The child psychiatric forensic evaluation of children and adolescents who are plaintiffs in civil lawsuits regarding their present and future damages from child maltreatment requires knowledge of current research findings on the short-term and long-term consequences of child maltreatment, evidence-based treatments for psychological trauma, and relevant professional guidelines, along with knowledge of the ethics and laws governing mental health expert practice and testimony in personal injury litigation. This article reviews current research and recommends an approach to these evaluations and expert testimony that is informed by current research findings, recently developed professional guidelines, and many years of professional experience.

During the Outreau case in France, 13 individuals were falsely accused of child sexual abuse and incarcerated. The author of this article testified as a psychiatric expert when the convictions were appealed. He explains how purposeful false statements by adults, inept expert witnesses, and the judicial assumption that children do not lie converged to create a tragic legal outcome. This article explains how psychiatric experts should conduct evaluations in cases of alleged child sexual abuse.

Forensic Evaluation and Testimony

Dramatic advances in the understanding of the neurobiological bases of human behavior have prompted excitement and controversy surrounding the ethical, legal, and social applications of this knowledge. The authors critically examine the promise and challenges of integrating genomic and neuroimaging techniques into legal settings. They suggest criteria for enhancing the viability of incorporating these data within a legal context and highlight several recent developments that may eventually allow genetic and neuroimaging evidence to meet these criteria and play a more prominent role in forensic science and law.

Research has established that children can make efforts to deceive others and that malingering or underperformance in psychiatric and psychological evaluations is common. Clinicians often resist the idea that children can successfully fake mental disorders and formal assessment for malingering is rare in clinical practice. The author suggests that screening tests be performed during the initial evaluation of all children to identify deceptive behavior. Children who behave in a suspect fashion and children who have known motivations to present as more pathologic than they are should be formally assessed with psychological techniques to rule out the presence of malingering.

When mental health experts express their opinions in testimony, reports, and articles in professional literature, it is expected that their statements will accurately reflect the current state of knowledge. Experts may disagree about the data that they collected. In some cases, however, disagreement occurs because an expert has employed a methodology that is far outside usual procedures or simply disregarded objective facts. When that occurs, the expert's opinions may be considered ridiculous. The author presents examples of ridiculous statements by mental health experts and provides suggestions for how a forensic practitioner might address ridiculous statements by mental health experts.

Training in Child and Adolescent Forensic Psychiatry

Exposure to child and adolescent forensic issues is limited in general psychiatry residency and child and adolescent psychiatry residency programs. There is no Graduate Medical Education Program for child and adolescent forensic psychiatry that is approved by the American Council on Graduate Medical Education (ACGME). Forensic psychiatry residency directors can create a child-focused forensic training opportunity that meets the needs of the ACGME program in forensic psychiatry. By creating didactic, clinical, and research experiences relevant to child and adolescent forensic psychiatric issues, this much-needed training can be provided to qualified psychiatrists.

To persuade a fact finder that a forensic opinion has a scientific basis, it is often useful to cite professional literature that supports one's opinions or procedures. If the admissibility of one's opinion is challenged in a Daubert hearing, citing literature is almost always required to support the claim that the expert's opinion relies on scientific facts or proceeds from scientific methodology. This annotated bibliography provides a sampling of articles that may be useful in bolstering testimony. The sample selected here is not comprehensive, but provides examples of literature that may be cited by forensic child and adolescent psychiatric experts.

RELATED INTEREST

Psychiatric Clinics of North America, Vol. 34, No. 1, March 2011
Prevention in Mental Health: Lifespan Perspective
Dilip V. Jeste, MD, and Carl C. Bell, MD, DLAPA, FACPsych, *Guest Editors*

THE CLINICS ARE NOW AVAILABLE ONLINE!

Access your subscription at:
www.theclinics.com

Foreword
"You Can't Handle
The Truth!"

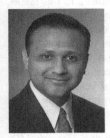

Harsh K. Trivedi, MD
Consulting Editor

The opportunity does not regularly present itself when I get to use the lay definition of a psychiatric term (particularly when the psychiatric definition of that term could be so far from how it is misused). However, not to waste this opportunity, let me begin by saying that the following two paragraphs represent the schizophrenic nature of forensic work in our field. By this, I mean that we have two very different populations within our clinical practitioners. We have those who could not be more distant from the knowledge and the comfort of dealing with such issues, while we have others who not only live in this world but also excel in this world and help many to find clarity in terms of what to do in these cases.

For many providers, their main exposure to court cases and to legal proceedings generally comes from the media. From the latest exciting John Grisham novel to watching movies such as *A Few Good Men*, the only image that comes up is that of a suspense-filled, highly intense, and anxiety-riddled scene. For the general practitioner who has been asked to testify in court, asked to provide a deposition, or even simply asked to discuss the ramifications of a potential legal issue, it is easy to relate how foreign some of these conversations can be from everyday clinical care. Yet, we practice in a world where we are faced with more patients and more families dealing with all types of legal issues, from custody battles, to truancy, to legal charges, and even to foreclosure.

For a handful of our colleagues, this is simply the world that they live in. They have trained in forensic psychiatry and are well versed in its nuances. They have been in many courts and they have dealt with many difficult cases. They have earnestly followed legal cases that have risen to the level of the Supreme Court. They have watched these trials discuss fundamental issues such as the ability of a minor to be tried as an adult. Some have even provided amicus briefs for these cases or testified as an expert witness for similar cases.

Child Adolesc Psychiatric Clin N Am 20 (2011) xiii–xiv
doi:10.1016/j.chc.2011.04.001
1056-4993/11/$ – see front matter © 2011 Elsevier Inc. All rights reserved.
childpsych.theclinics.com

This dichotomy belies the difficulty in creating a salient and meaningful issue of the clinics on this topic. I want to sincerely thank our guest editors, Bill Bernet and Bradley Freeman, for doing justice to meeting the needs of our entire readership. They have been able to compile an issue that balances the needs of both sets of providers. You will find articles that are helpful to those who are novices at legal issues as well as articles that will challenge and broaden the knowledge base of our most seasoned forensic experts. I would like to thank each of the wonderful contributors to this issue for sharing their expertise and for allowing us to have these very complex issues discussed in a very practical and clinically relevant manner. Whether you are the expert or whether you are propelled into these cases (sometimes unwillingly), it is my sincere hope that you will find this issue to be of great value to your clinical practice. From the wonderful line said by Jack Nicholson in *A Few Good Men*, let us hope that not only will you be able to handle the truth, but that you will also be able to help others discover the truth as it pertains to the children and families that we treat.

Harsh K. Trivedi, MD
Vanderbilt Psychiatric Hospital
1601 23rd Avenue South, Suite 1157
Nashville, TN 37212, USA

E-mail address:
harsh.k.trivedi@vanderbilt.edu

Preface

Forensic Psychiatry

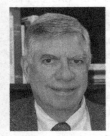 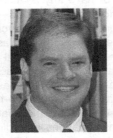

William Bernet, MD   Bradley W. Freeman, MD
Guest Editors

Child and adolescent psychiatrists encounter legal and administrative issues on a regular basis, even if they do not actively practice forensic psychiatry. For example, the child psychiatrist may be treating a child whose parents divorce, and suddenly both the child and his psychiatrist are thrust into the middle of an angry battle between the parents. Or, an adolescent psychiatrist may be treating a youngster who misbehaves in a serious manner and they both end up in juvenile court, the psychiatrist testifying with regard to her delinquent patient. Or, any physician may find himself a defendant in a medical malpractice lawsuit. Of course, child and adolescent psychiatrists who also specialize in and practice forensic psychiatry face these issues every day. This issue of *Child and Adolescent Psychiatric Clinics of North America* is intended for both the general clinician and the forensic specialist.

The theme of this issue of the *Clinics* is to look beyond the basics. In this issue, we have not attempted to reframe and rehash the fundamentals of child and adolescent forensic psychiatry, which have been thoroughly presented in previous issues of this journal and in basic textbooks. Instead, we have selected articles that address topics that are more focused and also important for both the clinician and the forensic specialist. For example, we do not explain how to conduct a forensic custody evaluation, but one article addresses the common but troublesome issue of what to do when the child of divorced parents refuses contact with one of the parents. We do not discuss how to conduct a pretrial forensic evaluation, but one article reviews the narrow topic of how behavioral genomics and neuroimaging might be used or misused in forensic evaluations.

This issue has five sections, and the first section addresses juvenile offenders. Gregg Dwyer and Elizabeth Letourneau summarize the history of treatment approaches for juveniles who sexually offend, and they describe contemporary, evidence-based protocols for treating these youths. David Siegel, a law professor, explains clearly how the US Supreme Court has emphasized in recent rulings that the sentencing of juvenile offenders should take their developmental immaturity into consideration. Jeff Bostic and Colby Brunt take on other topics—school bullying

Child Adolesc Psychiatric Clin N Am 20 (2011) xv–xvii
doi:10.1016/j.chc.2011.03.014
1056-4993/11/$ – see front matter © 2011 Elsevier Inc. All rights reserved.

and cyberbullying—that have received a great deal of attention in both general media and professional literature.

The second section pertains to child custody and visitation. Bradley Freeman addresses the behavioral symptom of contact refusal, that is, the situation when the child of divorced parents refuses to visit or have any relationship with one of the parents. Contact refusal is simply a behavior, not a diagnosis—like school refusal—and this article explains the differential diagnosis of that symptom. One of the several causes of contact refusal is parental alienation and Douglas Darnall, a forensic psychologist, explains the psychosocial treatment of parental alienation. He points out that children who manifest parental alienation are more easily treated when their condition is in its early stages rather than later, when it becomes severe and perhaps refractory. When divorced parents are impaired in some way—for example, because of a mental condition or substance abuse—forensic psychiatrists are sometimes asked to evaluate them and make recommendations regarding the arrangements for parenting time or visitation. Stephen Montgomery and David Street explain the principles for conducting these evaluations and making relevant recommendations to the court.

The third section of this issue relates to child maltreatment. Occasionally, child and adolescent forensic psychiatrists are asked to evaluate plaintiffs in civil lawsuits, who claim that they were physically or sexually abused. David Corwin and Brooks Keeshin review current research on the short-term and long-term effects of child abuse, and they explain how that research may inform the evaluations and expert testimony in those cases. Paul Bensussan, a forensic psychiatrist in France, provides a general account and his own personal involvement with an infamous case—the Outreau case—in which several individuals were accused of child sexual abuse. Bensussan helped the appellate court sort out which allegations were true and which were false, and he subsequently received the Legion d'honneur from the French government for his work as a forensic psychiatrist.

The fourth section pertains to specific features of forensic evaluation and testimony, which may be considered controversial. Michael Treadway and Joshua Buckholtz, who are neuroscientists, explore a fascinating issue that has confronted forensic practitioners in the last decade: the recent advances in behavioral genomics and neuroimaging. Treadway and Buckholtz explain how these cutting-edge scientific techniques might be both used and misused in legal settings. James Walker, a forensic neuropsychologist, tackles an interesting topic that has rarely been addressed in a systematic manner, that is, whether children malinger in psychiatric and psychological evaluations. William Bernet describes several situations in which mental health experts expressed opinions in a manner that was so flawed it could be considered ridiculous, and he explains what others might do when observing such a performance.

Finally, the last section addresses an extremely important topic, the training of psychiatrists who are interested in both child and adolescent psychiatry and forensic psychiatry. Charles Scott provides practical guidance for how a training director might organize a child and adolescent psychiatry forensic track within a one-year training program in forensic psychiatry. The final article—by Peter Ash and Paul O'Leary—is an annotated bibliography for the testifying child and adolescent psychiatrist. This will be helpful in training programs and also for any child and adolescent psychiatrist who is preparing to testify at a deposition or in court.

We hope that this issue of the *Clinics* will interest clinical practitioners as well as child and adolescent psychiatrists with extensive experience in the subspecialty of forensic psychiatry. The topics discussed in this issue are meant to be both informative and provocative—we aim to highlight the importance of child and adolescent forensic issues and the complex interactions of family systems and the legal system. We hope you enjoy this issue and that you are able to incorporate this material into your own practice.

William Bernet, MD

Bradley W. Freeman, MD

Department of Psychiatry
Vanderbilt University School of Medicine
1601 23rd Avenue South
Nashville, TN 37212, USA

E-mail addresses:
william.bernet@vanderbilt.edu (W. Bernet)
bradley.w.freeman@vanderbilt.edu (B.W. Freeman)

Juveniles Who Sexually Offend: Recommending a Treatment Program and Level of Care

R. Gregg Dwyer, MD, EdD[a,b,*], Elizabeth J. Letourneau, PhD[c]

KEYWORDS

- Juveniles • Sexual offending • Evaluation
- Risk assessment • Treatment

Sexual offending by juveniles has been a significant problem in the United States for many years. Based on national victimization data, approximately one-quarter (26.3%; n = 42,151) of single perpetrator rapes are committed by adolescents.[1] Based on 2008 national arrest data, adolescents account for 15% (n = 2505) of forcible rapes and 18% (n = 11,029) of sex offenses other than forcible rape and prostitution.[2] These figures are consistent with the study of sex crimes against children that estimated that adolescents commit 23% of all sex offenses, 4% of offenses against adults, 33% of offenses against all ages of children, and 40% of offenses against victims less than 6 years of age.[3] When minors are the victims, 35.6% had juvenile perpetrators, with 1 out of 8 offenders being younger than 12 years.[4] Police involvement in such cases increases significantly when juveniles who sexually offend are aged 12 to 14 years and then plateaus. Offenders in middle and late adolescence tend to be more likely to have victims who are teenagers rather than preteens.[4]

HISTORICAL ATTITUDES

From early on, juveniles who sexually offended were viewed as mini-adults in terms of offending cause and risk and, therefore, treatment approaches. This in part was

There was no financial support for this work. The authors have nothing to disclose.
[a] Forensic Psychiatry Program, Department of Psychiatry and Behavioral Sciences, Medical University of South Carolina, Charleston, SC, USA
[b] Sexual Behaviors Clinic and Lab, Department of Psychiatry and Behavioral Sciences, Medical University of South Carolina, Charleston, SC, USA
[c] Department of Psychiatry and Behavioral Sciences, Family Services Research Center, Medical University of South Carolina, Charleston, SC, USA
* Corresponding author. Forensic Psychiatry Program, Department of Psychiatry and Behavioral Sciences, 29-C Leinbach Drive, Charleston, SC 29407.
E-mail address: dwyer@musc.edu

Child Adolesc Psychiatric Clin N Am 20 (2011) 413–429
doi:10.1016/j.chc.2011.03.007
1056-4993/11/$ – see front matter © 2011 Elsevier Inc. All rights reserved.

because of the observation that some paraphilic adult offenders began offending during adolescence, which led to the misconception that unmodifiable, traitlike characteristics (eg, deviant arousal patterns) were at the root of all sexual offending.[4] Programs for juveniles originated in the late 1980s and early 1990s that essentially replicated adult treatment models. There was a belief that juveniles who committed sex offenses were destined to become adult sexual predators and therefore should be treated as adults in terms of treatment content and setting, with the latter often being a secure placement.

The 1993 Revised Report from the National Task Force on Juvenile Sexual Offending cemented the view that juveniles who sexually offend were predestined to become adult sex offenders. Thus, treatment was intended to facilitate control of (rather than elimination of) abusive behaviors.[5] It was assumed that treatment had to be sex offense specific and be conducted in groups composed entirely of youths who had sexually offended. At the time, confrontational approaches were common in adult programs and hence were also introduced with juveniles. Elimination of offense denial was a requirement for community placement and/or treatment completion. Programs often combined aspects of psychodynamic, cognitive, behavioral, and educational approaches, and others focused exclusively on addressing deviant arousal.[5] However, work on identification and breaking of the cycle of offending was a common goal. Again, this was an outgrowth of the adult approach that was based on a substance abuse treatment model. Duration of treatment of juveniles was generally expected to be 12 to 24 months and often in criminal justice or private residential settings.[5]

Since 1986, the Safer Society Press has published results from 9 sex offender treatment provider surveys.[6] These surveys provide a snapshot of clinical practices in the United States and (most recently) Canada, with results separated by client gender, age (adult, adolescent, child), and treatment setting (community based or residential). Based on these surveys and other reviews (eg, American Academy of Child and Adolescent Psychiatry[7]), cognitive-behavioral therapy within a relapse-prevention framework (CBT-RP) quickly became and remains the dominant theory on which treatment programs for juveniles who sexually offended were developed.

Thus, more than 85% of programs serving adolescent boys indicated that cognitive-behavioral theory was one of the primary theories guiding their programs, with relapse prevention the next most frequently endorsed theory, followed by psychosocial-educational theory. Consistent with these theories, which emphasize youth-level deficits as the primary drivers of juvenile sexual offending, treatment targets nearly always included social skills training, improving victim awareness and empathy, taking responsibility for the offense, problem solving, and intimacy/relationship skills building.

Treatment modalities have also included occasional use of medications such as antiandrogens and selective serotonin reuptake inhibitors, occasional individual psychodynamic therapy, and family therapy.[8]

Because of the numerous treatment targets and mix of treatment modalities that comprise typical programs, the duration of community-based treatment is 14 months and programs require an average of 182 hours for completion (excluding aftercare or booster sessions).[6] However, many of the individual youth deficits targeted by programs do not consistently map onto the treatment or criminogenic needs of these youth. For example, neither offender denial nor level of victim empathy predict recidivism, yet both are nearly universally targeted in treatment programs. Research on adults who have sexually offended suggests that the inclusion of noncriminogenic needs dilutes treatment effectiveness,[9] as does mismatching treatment dose with individual risk level.[10] One study showed that lower-risk adult sex offenders benefited to the same extent whether they completed 60 or 180 hours of treatment; thus briefer treatment is likely to be both clinically and cost effective relative to longer treatment of some offenders. Requiring the average juvenile client to complete 182 hours of community-based treatment across a 14-month time period virtually guarantees that most youth are receiving excessive treatment.

Another fundamental shortcoming of treatment approaches has been the one-size-fits-all approach, which is coupled with the use of the wrong size (ie, that of adults). The first mistake applies to adults as well in that sex offending is a behavior, not a diagnosis, and as such has multiple causes. Effective management to include treatment requires identification, when possible, of the most relevant motivators of the problem behavior for a given youth. The second failure is in applying approaches designed and developed for adults, who are physically, cognitively, emotionally, and socially different than juveniles who still are developing across the aforementioned domains until their late teen years to early 20s.

FACTORS ASSOCIATED WITH JUVENILE SEXUAL OFFENDING

The strongest evidence for factors associated with youth behavior problems comes from longitudinal studies that prospectively follow cohorts from birth or early childhood through adulthood. The general delinquency literature has benefited from several such longitudinal studies conducted during the past 25 years.[11] Data from these projects have been used to identify factors consistently associated with general delinquency (see reviews by Elliott,[12] Henggeler,[13] Huizinga,[14] and Loeber and colleagues[15]). Risk and protective factors occur across the ecological systems in which youth are embedded. As summarized by Schoenwald and Rowland,[16] favorable attitudes toward antisocial behavior contribute to, and intelligence protects against, delinquency at the individual youth level; high family conflict contributes to, and attachment to parents protects against, risk at the family level; association with deviant peers contributes to, and bonding with prosocial peers protects against, risk at the peer level; dropout contributes to, and commitment to schooling protects against, risk at the school level; and high disorganization contributes to, and a strong indigenous support network protects against, risk at the community level.[16]

Similar factors seem to be associated with both general and sexual delinquency. For example, using data from the longitudinal Pittsburgh Youth Study,[15] van Wijk and colleagues[17] compared youth who committed violent sexual offenses with youth who committed other violent offenses. The groups had nonsignificant differences on 64 of 66 (97%) factors, suggesting broad overlap. Likewise, in a recent meta-analysis, Seto and Lalumière[18] compared results from 59 studies that included both juveniles who had sexually offended and juveniles with nonsexual offenses. The 2 groups were statistically similar on 21 of 37 (57%) factors that were examined. However, there were numerous factors on which the 2 groups reliably differed, suggesting that pathways for juveniles who sexually offend, or for at least some of these youth, diverge from those of juveniles who are nonsexually delinquent. In particular, the between-groups differences with the largest effects sizes were for atypical sexual interests and history of child sexual abuse victimization, which were more common among youth who had sexual offenses, and criminal history, antisocial associations, and substance use, which were more common among youth who had nonsexual offenses. The investigators speculated that atypical sexual interests (eg, sexual interest in prepubescent children or coercive sex with peers or adults) motivates some youth who commit sexual offenses and "antisocial tendencies influence an adolescent's willingness to act upon this motivation."[18]

DEVELOPMENTAL FACTORS

How atypical sexual interest might initially develop in youth and how it might be maintained for the minority of youth who continue sexually offending in adulthood is an understudied area of research. Sexual development runs along a continuum from normalcy to deviancy, with inappropriate behaviors not being definite predictors of sexual deviancy and, for juveniles, there is no clear line between normal and pathologic.[19] During early adolescence, youth have an increased curiosity and concern about their own bodies, appearance, and self-image, an increase in sexual fantasies, an increase in masturbation, and sometimes a sense of shame and guilt with the adults in their lives occasionally experiencing discomfort and anxiety.[19]

Middle adolescence is marked by an increase in sexual energy; the start of casual relationships; coital and noncoital interactions, which can be exploratory, promiscuous, or exploitive; a denial of risk to include pregnancy and sexually transmitted diseases; and the struggle to balance personal needs with daily demands.[19] By late adolescence, physical maturation is complete, sexual behavior is more expressive, less exploitive and more mutual, their psychosocial identify is in less flux, they have developed moral and ethical standards of behavior, and they have a social network to support independence from caregivers.[19]

Sources of unhealthy sexual behaviors include reactive modeling, premature sexualization, pervasive conduct problems, interpersonal relationship deficits, and wide range impairment leading to opportunistic behaviors, which frequently are isolated and time limited.[19] A growing body of research implicates biologic causes for adult pedophilia. For example, relative to other sex offenders and nonoffenders, pedophilic men are more likely to be left-handed, are shorter, and have lower intelligence quotients (IQs).[20] However, support for biologic causes has not emerged for juvenile offenders. For example, in their meta-analysis, Seto and Lalumière[18] reported that juveniles who had sexually offended and those who had nonsexually offended were similar with respect to general intelligence, verbal and performance IQs, and history of neurologic anomalies.[18]

There is no universal, or even dominant, explanation for juvenile sex offending. The population is heterogeneous and it is likely that multiple pathways to juvenile sexual offending exist. This heterogeneity requires treatment to be tailored to the individual youth, thus necessitating a comprehensive evaluation to identify behavior cause, risk, and, ultimately, treatment targets.

PSYCHIATRIC EVALUATION

Evaluations are conducted for treatment planning, risk assessment, management level determination, and to address nonsexual offending issues.[19,20] The evaluation process continues throughout the treatment process and, in some cases, youth become more forthcoming in time, as a therapeutic relationship is built. Moreover, the contingencies of the preadjudication investigations and adjudication procedures do not lend themselves to complete honesty.[21] Preadjudication assessments present particular challenges, given that no assessment instrument or combination of instruments can help determine guilt or innocence, but nevertheless often are used to sway judges' adjudication decisions.[22]

Given the seriousness of decisions based at least in part on assessment outcomes (eg, whether youth remain at home or within secure facilities; whether youth will be subjected to registration and notification procedures), national standards for conducting assessments should be available. They are not. The American Academy of Child and Adolescent Psychiatry published practice parameters in 1999 and, although up-to-date at the time, much of the guideline has become outdated with advances in knowledge.[7] The Association for the Treatment of Sexual Abusers has such standards for adults but has not yet produced separate juvenile standards.[23] The International Association for the Treatment of Sexual Offenders has a brief, 4-page summary of recommendations. In this vacuum, several states have enacted sex offender management boards that developed their own idiosyncratic evaluation, risk assessment, and treatment requirements for juveniles. Despite a lack of national standards, it is generally accepted that juvenile sex offending is a behavior, not a diagnosis, and a behavior that is variably influenced by a heterogeneous mix of risk and protective factors. Consequently, evaluations must broadly address a wide range of potentially relevant factors to best determine characteristics that might be implicated in the cause and/or maintenance of sexual offending in a given youth.

Evaluations are informed by 3 categories of information: (1) clinical information including review of records, interview(s) of the youth being evaluated, their parents/caregivers, and collateral source interviews; (2) self-reported and parent/caregiver-reported psychometric assessment instruments; and (3) physiologic testing. Record reviews should include, when applicable, police reports, victim statements, protective service reports, probation reports, and medical, corrections, court, hospital and school records.[6,21,22] Interviews with parents or other caregivers should always be included in assessment procedures involving juvenile patients. Additional collateral sources include extended family members, current teachers, current and prior therapists, and the youth's physicians. For intrafamilial sex offense cases, interviews with victims might also be warranted, but only if the victim has no objection and with a therapist available for the victim.[21,24]

Clinical Interviews

Interviews with youth and their parents/caregivers should be systematic and thorough but flexible, with the understanding that denial and minimization of inappropriate behaviors are normative for juveniles.[6,21,25] Interview topics for youth and caregivers should include developmental, family, educational, social, general medical, psychiatric, victimization, substance use, criminal, and sexual histories and a mental status examination.[6,21,26,27] The youth's developmental history focuses on maternal health[6,21,26,27] such as infections, trauma, medication use and substance abuse during pregnancy, and birth complications.[6,21,26] In addition, a description of milestones attainment, family interactions, and peer relationships is important.[21,27] Developmental issues, past experiences, and current functioning all affect treatment recommendations.[21,26]

Family history should address the parents' psychosocial histories, disciplinary methods, nature and degree of support, and extent and quality of displays of affection, aggression, love, and sexuality.[6,21] Educational history addresses cognitive ability and academic performance through the use of grade reports and school psychological testing.[6,26,27] Criminal history includes not only sexual offenses but all arrests, convictions, commitments/incarcerations,[6,26] use of a weapon, and animal cruelty.[6]

Sexual history addresses knowledge, sexual identity, orientation, gender, self-perception, fantasy, behavior experience, aggression,[21,26] desire and/or attempt to change,[21] and genital anomalies and injury.[21,27] Sexual experience is defined broadly as dating, kissing, petting, masturbation, genital intercourse, opposite and same-sex contacts and exposure to and use of sexually explicit material.[6,21,25,27] Internet exposure to sexual material, exposure via other media (eg, sexually explicit magazines), and more recent technology-driven methods for sending/receiving sexually explicit material or communications (eg, sexual content chat room use and so-called sexting) should also be explored. Evaluation should include assessment of potential sexual aggression, which can be ascertained by descriptions of past sex offenses, including victim profiles and context of offenses.[6,21]

The mental status examination[6,26] is used to screen for psychopathology; organicity; basic cognitive dysfunction; personality disorders; substance abuse; defense mechanisms; coping skills; and suicide history, risk, and current ideations/plans.[6] Assessment of the youth's own victimization experiences should include physical and sexual abuse, neglect, and exposure to family sexuality or other developmentally inappropriate sexual activity.[6,21,25,26] The medical history is intended to identify not only general medical diagnosis,[6,19,26,27] but also level of sexual maturity, presence of sexually transmitted disease, and psychiatric symptoms.[6,19]

Psychological Testing and Data Collection Instruments

There is no single test or assessment instrument for identifying inappropriate sexual behavior or future risk.[6,21] However, there are a wide variety of psychometric assessment instruments that can inform evaluations. These instruments typically rely on youth self-report, although a few also include parent report. These self-report and parent-report instruments can be used to assess general mental health issues that seem more common among juveniles who sexually offend, such as anxiety, general delinquency concerns, and factors that seem more specifically related to sexual offending, such as atypical sexual interests, youth's own victimization history, and social isolation. Other instruments commonly included in comprehensive evaluations, despite a lack of evidence relating them to offense initiation or maintenance, assess anger control, general or victim empathy, attachment, attention-deficit and impulsivity disorders, self-esteem, and other mental health problems (eg, depression) and personality traits.[21]

The parent-reported Child Behavior Checklist[28] and the corresponding Youth Self-Report[29] assess internalizing (eg, anxiety, depression) and externalizing (eg, conduct disorder) mental health symptoms. These instruments are well validated and considered among the best for assessing youth mental health functioning.[30] The Self-Report of Delinquency[31] is regarded as one of the best-validated measures of delinquency[32] and includes items assessing a range of delinquent behaviors (eg, assault, theft, sexual offenses) across a range of settings (eg, school, home, community).

Atypical sexual interests can be assessed with the Adolescent Sexual Interest Card Sort.[33,34] This instrument consists of 64 vignettes describing sexual acts or situations that youth rate on a 5-point scale from "really turns me off sexually" to "really turns me on sexually." Adequate test-retest and internal consistency have been reported, although concurrent validity was not supported, in that self-report results did not correlate with physiologically assessed sexual interest results.[34] A more comprehensive self-report instrument is the Multiphasic Sex Inventory II Adolescent Male (Female) Form.[35] This instrument assesses several paraphilias, conduct disorder, aggressive behavior, substance use, attention-deficit/hyperactivity disorder, and other potentially relevant comorbid problems.[35] The developers provide scale norms and reported that internal consistency ranged from good to excellent for the 4 primary scales. A new instrument that includes both youth and parent report is the Adolescent Clinical Sexual Behavior Inventory (ACSBI).[36,37] The ACSBI is a 45-item questionnaire that measures inappropriate or concerning sexual behaviors and includes subscales specifically assessing divergent sexual interests and sexual risk/misuse. The ACSBI has shown adequate reliability and validity with nonabused and with sexually abused youth, of whom a significant percentage reported engaging in sexually abusive acts.[36,37]

Youth victimization histories are comprehensively assessed with semistructured interviews[38] rather than paper-and-pencil self-report instruments. However, the effects of trauma can be assessed using such instruments as the Children's Impact of Traumatic Events Scale-Revised.[39]

Physiologic Testing

Physiologic testing can be used to identify endocrine abnormalities that can lead to mood, anxiety, and sexual disorder symptoms; attention deficits and impulsivity; and atypical sexual interest or sexual arousal patterns. For atypical sexual interest or arousal patterns, methods include visual reaction time (VRT) measurement, penile plethysmography, and polygraphy. VRT assessment is an objective measure of a person's time viewing photographs of clothed male and female children, teens, and adults.[6,23] Approximately one-third of male adolescent treatment programs use VRT.[6] Fischer and Smith[40] conducted a review of one such VRT system, the Abel Assessment for Sexual Interests in Paraphilias, the predecessor of the Abel Assessment for Sexual Interest (AASI), and reported only minimal evidence of its validity and reliability for use with adults and none for use with adolescents. In a retrospective comparison study of VRT, results of adolescent boys with child victims compared with a group with other inappropriate sexual behaviors, Abel and his colleagues[41] found the VRT system able to differentiate the 2 groups. Worling[42] compared 2 self-report instruments and a VRT method for assessing sexual arousal among male adolescents who had admitted committing contact sexual offenses.[42] The VRT and self-report methods were all able to distinguish adolescents who had male child victims from those adolescents who did not, but none could differentiate between adolescents with female child victims from those with other victim groups.[42] Fanniff and Becker[43] recommended further research for AASI use with adolescents and, if its results are included in an evaluation report, there should also be a note describing the limited research literature support.

Penile plethysmography (PPG) measures sexual arousal by assessing change in penile tumescence in response to sexual stimuli.[44] Except in cases of serious or frequent sexual aggression behaviors, this test is recommended more frequently for use with adults than adolescents because of concerns about the limited empirical support, consent issues, and exposure of youths to sexually explicit material.[25,45,46] Consequently, PPG is used by far fewer treatment programs (9%) than is VRT.[6] The PPG has been documented to have discriminatory power when used with adolescents in some settings. In particular, as with VRT, there is evidence that PPG testing discriminates between youth with male, as opposed to female-only victims.[47,48] There is just 1 published examination of the predictive validity of the PPG when used with juveniles. In this study by Clift and colleagues,[47] posttreatment arousal to male and female children regardless of context (forced or not) and posttreatment inability to suppress arousal to male and female children under suppress instructions correlated with sexual offense recidivism across a 6-year follow-up period. The researchers did not find that pretreatment arousal predicted recidivism.

Not a single study of PPG or VRT has been published that included a nonoffending sample of youth. This serious gap significantly curtails generalizations that can be made about the results, or even the meaning, of VRT and PPG testing results. Moreover, distinguishing between youth aroused to boys versus youth aroused to girls seems to be of limited usefulness especially given that this information can be ascertained from other sources. The predictive validity results found by Clift and colleagues[47] are encouraging but need to be replicated with additional studies.

Several studies have shown that polygraph testing increases the *rates* of disclosures by adults[49,50] and juveniles[51] who have sexually offended. However, the *accuracy* of such disclosures is almost completely unknown. Of 3 types of postconviction polygraph examinations, data suggest that only 1, the specific issue examination, likely detects lies at significantly greater than chance levels, although such detection remains imperfect.[52] Data do not support the more common full disclosure and monitoring or maintenance examinations. Concerns have been raised about subjecting youth to testing that lacks even basic psychometric support.[43] In particular, polygraph testing might induce false disclosures by youth trying to pass the test. The presence of such demand characteristics seems likely, given that 50% of US adolescent treatment programs use 1 or more types of polygraph examinations, and a high percentage (eg, 27% of community programs for boys) require youth to pass full-disclosure polygraph examinations before they are successfully discharged from treatment.

RISK ASSESSMENT

A growing area of clinical practice involves the assessment of juvenile sexual and nonsexual recidivism risk. Such risk assessments are used to inform decisions regarding sentencing and postsentencing requirements (eg, registration and notification requirements), appropriate treatment setting (eg, community based vs residential), treatment intensity, and supervision requirements.[53,54] The 2002 and 2009 Safer Society surveys included questions about the use of sexual recidivism risk assessment instruments. Three instruments are in wide use, including the Estimate of Risk of Adolescent Sexual Offense Recidivism (ERASOR),[55] Juvenile Sex Offender Assessment Protocol-II (J-SOAP-II)[56] and Juvenile Sexual Offense Recidivism Risk Assessment Tool-II (JSORRAT-II) (Epperson DL, Ralston CA, Fowers D, et al. Development of a sexual offense recidivism risk assessment tool-II [JSORRAT-II]. Ames [IA]: University of Iowa; 2005. Unpublished manuscript).

The ERASOR is a checklist of 25 risk factors intended to assist clinical estimates regarding short-term risk for sexual recidivism.[57] Although not intended to provide a single score but rather a relative ranking of low, moderate, or high risk, use of a total score manufactured by summing the individual item scores has been observed. The JSORRAT-II is a 12-item actuarial instrument designed to assess for risk of violence in juveniles who have sexually offended (Epperson DL, Ralston CA, Fowers D, et al. Development of a sexual offense recidivism risk assessment tool-II [JSORRAT-II]. Ames [IA]: University of Iowa; 2005. Unpublished manuscript). Item scoring is objective and criterion-based and a total score is created by summing item scores. The J-SOAP-II is a checklist of 25 risk factors designed to assess risk of sexual and general delinquency. The J-SOAP-II provides a total score with which to estimate recidivism risk, 4 additional scale scores addressing sexual drive/sexual preoccupation, impulsive/antisocial behavior, clinical/treatment, and community adjustment and 2 summary scores for static and dynamic factors.

Most studies that examined the psychometric properties of these risk assessment instruments report evidence of adequate to excellent reliability for instrument scale and total scores. However, predictive validity results have varied markedly across studies. Many findings in support of predictive validity have been published by the tests' authors. For example, Epperson and colleagues (Epperson DL, Ralston CA, Fowers D, et al. Development of a sexual offense recidivism risk assessment tool-II [JSORRAT-II]. Ames [IA]: University of Iowa; 2005. Unpublished manuscript) reported excellent predictive validity for the JSORRAT-II for sexual recidivism. In a retrospective study, Worling[57] reported that the ERASOR total score significantly discriminated youth with single versus multiple sex offense charges. Likewise, Prentky and colleagues[56] reported that the J-SOAP-II total score significantly predicted sexual recidivism for high-risk preadolescents and high-risk adolescents. Findings from external reviews have been mixed. In the only other publication examining predictive validity of the JSORRAT,[58] the total score failed to predict sexual or any other type of posttreatment recidivism. In the 2 published studies that examined the predictive validity of the ERASOR, the total score failed to predict sexual or other recidivism[54] in one study and significantly predicted sexual recidivism in the other.[53]

Of the 4 published studies that examined the predictive validity of the J-SOAP-II total score, 2 found support,[53,59] whereas 2 did not.[58,60] It has been suggested that disparate results might be attributable to differences in study samples (eg, residential treatment samples vs criminal justice samples) and more generally to the heterogeneity of juveniles who sexually offend. For example, Rajlic and Gretton[53] analyzed results separately for youth with evidence of sexual plus nonsexual delinquency compared with youth with sex-limited delinquency. ERASOR and J-SOAP-II total scores significantly predicted sexual recidivism in the sex-limited group but failed to do so in the mixed delinquency group, even though youth in the latter group were more likely to sexually reoffend. Thus, as noted by those investigators, offending pathways and motivations that underlie sexual recidivism might be more complex for youth with multiple indicators of delinquency than for youth whose delinquency is limited to sex offenses.

No instrument is characterized by consistently supportive predictive validity findings, and virtually all investigators, and especially instrument developers, have cited a need for ongoing research and warned against the misuse of instrument scores.[56] Moreover, when making treatment recommendations, "clinicians should carefully acknowledge current limitations in their ability to predict adolescent sexual reoffending."[54] In particular, using such scores to determine whether youth should be subjected to long-term legal requirements such as registration or public notification is unwarranted.[61–63]

MATCHING TREATMENT TO PSYCHOSOCIAL NEEDS

When evaluations indicate treatment needs and/or recidivism concerns, interventions to reduce risk of harm should be made available to youths and their families. The history of treatment approaches for adolescents has been presented and, as noted earlier, most programs are based on a single, CBT-RP conceptualization of youth treatment needs. What is the present situation? There has been a growing awareness and, in turn, a shift in development and conduct of treatment to empirically supported methods.

As subsequently reviewed, family-focused interventions have the strongest evidence base for treating juveniles who have sexually offended. Thus, to improve treatment effectiveness and provide appropriate treatment dose, programs should move toward more family-focused services and should target treatment factors more closely related to youth recidivism risk. There is some evidence that programs are moving in this direction. For example, most juvenile treatment programs surveyed in 2009 included family support networks as a core treatment target and this percentage increased from the prior year's survey. Thus, 94% of US community-based programs addressed family support networks, up from 86% in the 2002 survey.[6,64] One empirically supported program (reviewed subsequently) has changed in the course of 22 years to emphasize family involvement, to match treatment intensity to estimated youth risk level, and to reduce or eliminate some treatment components (eg, discussion of individual youth sexual interests is now limited to individual rather than group sessions). As a result, the average treatment length has declined from 24 months to 16 months.[65] However, on average, US community-based programs currently included just 1 hour of family therapy per month, compared with 6 hours of group treatment and 3 hours of individual treatment per month.[6]

Clinically efficacious and cost effective treatment needs to attend closely to factors that contribute to the maintenance of juvenile sexual offending (ie, factors associated with recidivism such as general delinquency and atypical sexual interests) and avoid apparently irrelevant factors (eg, neither victim empathy nor distorted cognitions about coercive sex or sex with children distinguished between groups nor do these factors predict recidivism). Moreover, youth who commit sexual offenses are heterogeneous and many are not easily characterized as generally delinquent or having atypical sexual interests. Thus, interventions must be flexible to address the specific factors that seem related to a given child's sexual offending behavior. For example, perhaps a teenager experienced sexual abuse when younger, developed anxiety, and became socially isolated. His offense could involve a neighborhood child with whom he is friends because he is unable to make same-age friends. Treatment of this youth would focus on developing appropriate social and dating skills. A different youth might be poorly supervised by his parents, thus providing opportunities to view inappropriate pornographic materials online and to associate with other poorly supervised and delinquent youth, with whom he commits a variety of delinquent behaviors, including a sexual offense. Treatment of this youth would need to focus on establishing consistent adult supervision and monitoring, developing clear family rules around pornography, healthy dating and sexual behaviors, and dissociating the youth from delinquent peers and increasing his association with prosocial peers.

Multisystemic Therapy

Henggeler and colleagues[46,66] have developed an intervention paradigm based on social ecological theory: Multisystemic Therapy (MST). MST is an evidence-based, home-based, and community-based treatment model originally developed and empirically validated for ethnically diverse populations of youths presenting with juvenile delinquency and their families. MST has several characteristics that make it particularly appropriate for the treatment of juveniles who have sexually offended. First, the home-based approach increases access to care for high-risk youth and families. Second, by intervening in the home and community, the MST therapist can observe and more effectively resolve barriers to safety (eg, youths' rooms can be examined for inappropriate sexual materials; problems with family sleeping arrangements can be identified and corrected, such as boys and girls sharing rooms or youths sharing mattresses), and adult supervision and monitoring of youth can be examined in situ. Third, MST is uniquely suited to address the multiple risk factors for delinquency and sexual offending because of its flexibility.

MST is not a typical, standardized, one-size-fits-all intervention in which the therapist follows a set of prearranged tasks in a time-limited sequence. Instead, therapists begin by conducting a multisystemic assessment of the cause of the problem behavior and then, based on this assessment, tailoring interventions to each family to best address the identified problem behaviors. Whereas traditional delinquency interventions typically target individual child factors as described earlier, MST interventions are directed toward individuals, families, peers, and (as needed) individuals in other systems that are involved in the identified problem, such as teachers and probation officers. Therefore, MST interventions can flexibly address the particular factors across systems that contribute to sexual offending and general delinquency for each adolescent and family. To accomplish this, MST draws on a variety of evidence-based interventions as part of a menu of intervention choices that can be used depending on the individual presentation of the youth. Within this flexible approach, treatment fidelity monitoring is well established and high MST fidelity has been shown to be related to better treatment outcome.[67]

Multisystemic Therapy for Problem Sexual Behaviors

Multisystemic Therapy for Problem Sexual Behaviors (MST-PSB) was adapted from MST. The overriding goals of MST-PSB and MST are to empower parents with the skills and resources needed to address youth behavior problems and to empower adolescents to cope with familial and extrafamilial problems. Treatment strategies derived from pragmatic family therapies, behavioral parent training, and cognitive-behavioral therapy are used to directly address intrapersonal (eg, cognitive problem solving), familial (eg, inconsistent discipline, low monitoring, family conflict), and extra-familial (eg, association with deviant peers and school difficulties) factors that are associated with serious antisocial behavior, including sexual offending. Because different factors are relevant for different youths and their families, MST interventions are individualized and flexible.

The adaptation of MST for youth problem sexual behaviors (MST-PSB)[68] enhances standard MST by addressing aspects of the social ecology that are functionally related to youth sexual delinquency. These adaptations include protocols to address (1) youth and caregiver denial about the offense, (2) safety planning to minimize the youth's access to potential victims, and (3) promotion of age-appropriate and normative social experiences with peers. Improved caregiver discipline intended to discourage youth contact with antisocial peers is an important mediator of MST-PSB treatment effectiveness.[69]

Three randomized clinical trials provide evidence of the effectiveness of MST-PSB[63,70,71] and emphasize the importance of family factors in attaining such positive outcomes.[69] Across studies, sexual recidivism rates, nonsexual recidivism rates, or proxies for recidivism (ie, sexual behavior problems and self-reported delinquency) were significantly lower for youth treated in the MST-PSB condition than in control conditions. In addition, costly out-of-home placements were greatly reduced. Results from the most recent trial indicated that treatment outcomes were mediated by care-giver discipline and negative peers. Thus, as caregivers became more effective at disciplining their youth, and as youth reduced their association with negative peers, treatment effects were enhanced.[69]

MST-PSB is a high-intensity approach. Providers carry low caseloads and work directly with families, schools, or other key parts of the social ecology in vivo. This level of intensity is expensive and is not always necessary for all youth with problem sexual behaviors. MST-PSB might be best reserved for high-need cases, cases in which out-of-home placement is a risk, in emergent circumstances or in the event of deterioration during less intensive treatment, or at certain key junctures in treatment such as imme-diately before and after family reunification.

Sexual Abuse: Family Education and Treatment

The Sexual Abuse: Family Education and Treatment (SAFE-T) program was initiated in the mid-1980s, when concern about the treatment needs of juveniles who sexually offend was just beginning to crystallize into specialized treatment programs. Unlike programs based on adult treatment, the SAFE-T program was developed from the ground up, with a youth-developmental perspective that emphasized not only the individual-level needs of youth but also the strengths and needs of their families. Thus, although treatment includes common specialized targets such as sex offense prevention planning, deviant arousal reduction, cognitive restructuring, and victim empathy, there also is a strong family treatment component that emphasizes enhanced family relationships. Frequent targets of family therapy include "marital discord, parental rejection of the offender, physical discipline and verbal aggression."[24] Youth receive a mix of group, individual, and family treatment that in recent years has lasted about 16 months.[65]

Worling and colleagues[65] have published 2 treatment outcome studies, the first presenting 10-year follow-up results and the second presenting 20-year follow-up results. To our knowledge, these represent the longest prospective follow-up studies of youth treated with a specialized juvenile sex offender intervention. The investigators compared youth who completed at least 10 months of treatment (n = 58) with a comparison group of youth referred only for assessment, referred for assessment and treatment but who refused treatment, and referred for assessment and treatment but who dropped out of treatment before 10 months (n = 90).[55]

Although not randomly assigned to groups, comparisons on numerous factors indicated that youth were comparable on relevant variables such as demographic characteristics (eg, age at assessment, socioeconomic status), offense characteristics (eg, prior charges), victim characteristics (eg, gender, relationship to offender), or on any of several instrument scores that assessed delinquency, aggression, social problems, psychopathology, family characteristics, and so on. Results from both studies indicated that, relative to comparison youth, treated youth had significantly fewer subsequent charges for sexual, nonsexual violent, nonviolent, or any criminal reoffense. Because many of the youth in the comparison sample received at least some treatment from external agencies or the SAFE-T program (67%), these results not only support a general treatment effect for the SAFE-T program but also suggest that it has incremental validity beyond that of other programs in which youth were treated.

One caveat to these studies is that treatment dropouts were moved from the treatment group to the comparison group. Some have argued that, when analyzing clinical results, participants should be retained in their original group, regardless of whether they completed (or even changed) treatment. In randomization trials, this is termed intention-to-treat analysis and is used to preserve the original randomization.[72] In a reanalysis of Worling and Curwen's[55] 10-year follow-up data, dropouts were retained in the treatment group, with the effect of greatly reducing between-groups differences in sexual recidivism rates.[73] The effect of a similar change on the 20-year data has not been reported.

Cognitive-Behavioral Therapy for Adolescent Sex Offenders

Cognitive-Behavioral Therapy for Adolescent Sex Offenders (CBT-ASO) is an intervention that includes an equal focus on adolescents and their caregivers. The structure and execution of this intervention protocol are grounded in behavioral and social learning theory models and embrace several basic behavioral science principles for helping adolescents in trouble. Although some of the exercises and treatment modules focus on sexual behavior, much of the basic program structure and general principles focus more on improving behavior, increasing self-control, and parenting in general. These goals are relevant to both sexual and nonsexual behavior, and recognize that the problems of youth with illegal sexual behavior are not solely, or often even mostly, sexual in nature. The protocol engages parents or caregivers in every module and session and is based on social learning, and ecological and behavioral theory. The core principles include positive reinforcement for desired behaviors/cognitions; encouraging social involvement with prosocial peers and discouraging contact with negative peers; encouraging investment in school and grades; engagement in prosocial activities; setting clear expectations; and encouraging parental support and engagement, supervision and monitoring, and parent-child communication.

CBT-ASO is thematically similar to the well-established and evidence-based Cognitive-Behavioral Therapy for Children with Sexual Behavior Problems (CBT-CSBP),[74,75] and was developed by the same group of researchers. CBT-ASO has been evaluated in an unpublished 15-year follow-up study. The study was one of the few follow-up studies of adolescent sex offenders to monitor for future child welfare sex abuse perpetration as well as criminal justice outcomes. Approximately 3% of program completers had a future sex crime arrest or perpetration report to child welfare (M. Chaffin, personal communication, October 2, 2010).

SUMMARY

The treatment of juveniles who have committed sex offenses has evolved from the ill-conceived application of adult sex offender methods without consideration for developmental, etiologic, or risk differences to an evidence-based, holistic approach with consideration of individual recidivism risk. Although still evolving and in need of methodologically sound longitudinal studies, there has been significant progress toward facilitating the healthy development of youths with problem sexual behavior histories. As inflammatory labels such as juvenile super-predator are relegated to their rightful place as myths, as methods of evaluation focus on the collection of data empirically supported to identify protective and risk factors and appropriate targets for treatment and management, a change can be made toward a family-focused model prompting healthy growth with less stigma, while protecting the youth in treatment and those in the community around them.[76]

Caution is mandated, given that the current reliance on risk-assessment instruments far outweighs the empirically established capabilities of these instruments. The available methods are few and the data virtually equal in support of their value and against their use in the context of legal proceedings, community notification, and registration and confinement decisions. The methods to evaluate risk are still problematic, but that should not stymie our application of treatments known to be effective.

Juveniles who have sexually offended are not a homogeneous population and, consequently, treatment and management methods must maintain flexibility to accommodate the variety of issues. The one-size-fits-all approach is clearly inadequate as a system response and may cause harm to some subjected to treatment settings or methods not applicable to their constellation of needs. Sexual offending is a behavior and not a diagnosis. Now that the field has identified, with supporting data, at least some risk factors of reoffending and has developed and tested treatment interventions with successful outcomes, systems must be modified to use what works. A small but growing body of evidence suggests that promising treatments for juveniles who have sexually offended are comprehensive, flexible, and family focused.

Future efforts should focus on developing up-to-date national standards for evaluations, longitudinal research to identify risk and protective factors, and empirically rigorous treatment outcomes studies. As the United States Supreme Court concluded in considering the constitutionality of applying the death penalty in cases involving offenses when the defendant was still a youth, adolescents have a "susceptibility to immature and irresponsible behavior," and they a have a "vulnerability and comparative lack of control over their immediate surroundings."[77] The Court's opinion also noted that, because youth "still struggle to define their identity," "even a heinous crime" is not "evidence of irretrievably depraved character."[77] Given that adolescents are still developing in every facet, the opportunity to foster a healthy path must be seized, customized to the needs of individual youths and their families, and without unnecessary obstacles to their becoming productive members of society.

REFERENCES

1. United States Department of Justice, Bureau of Justice Statistics. Criminal victimization in the United States, 2005 statistical tables. Washington DC; December 2006. Report No. NCJ 215244.
2. United States Department of Justice, Federal Bureau of Investigation. Crime in the United States, 2008. September 2009. Available at: http://www.fbi.gov/ucr/cius2008/about/index.html. Accessed January 22, 2010.
3. Snyder HN. Sexual assault of young children as reported to law enforcement: victim, incident, and offender characteristics. NCJ 182990. Washington, DC: Office of Justice Programs, US Department of Justice; 2000. p. 1–14.
4. Finkelhor D, Ormrod R, Chaffin M. Juveniles who commit sex offenses against minors, NCJ 227763. Washington, DC: US Department of Justice Office of Justice Programs, Office of Juvenile Justice and Delinquency Prevention; 2009. p. 1–11.
5. National Adolescent Perpetrators Network (NAPN). The revised report from the National Task Force on Juvenile Sexual Offending. Juv Fam Court J 1993;44:5–91.
6. McGrath R, Cumming G, Burchard B, et al. Current practices and emerging trends in sexual abuser management: the Safer Society 2009 North American Survey. Brandon (VT): Safer Society Press; 2010.
7. American Academy of Child and Adolescent Psychiatry. Practice parameters for the assessment and treatment of children and adolescents who are sexually abusive of others. J Am Acad Child Adolesc Psychiatry 1999;38(Suppl 12): 55S–76S.
8. Becker JV. Offenders: characteristics and treatment. Future Child 1994;4(2): 176–97.
9. Hanson RK, Bourgon G, Helmus L, et al. A meta-analysis of the effectiveness of treatment for sexual offenders: risk, need and responsivity. Public Safety Canada; 2009. Available at: http://www.publicsafety.gc.ca/res/cor/rep/_fl/2009-01-trt-so-eng.pdf. Accessed April 13, 2011.
10. Beech A, Fisher D, Beckett R. Step 3: An evaluation of the Prison Sex Offender Treatment Programme: a report for the Home Office by the STEP team. London: Home Office Information Publications Group; 1998. Available at: http://rds.homeoffice.gov.uk/rds/pdfs/occ-step3.pdf. Accessed April 13, 2011.
11. Loeber R, Farrington DP, Stouthamer-Loeber M, et al. Antisocial behavior and mental health problems. Explanatory factors in childhood and adolescence. London: Lawrence Erlbaum; 1998.
12. Elliott DS. Serious violent offenders: onset, developmental course, and termination – The American Society of Criminology 1993 President Address. Criminology 1994;32:1–21.
13. Henggeler SW. The development of effective drug abuse services for youth. In: Egertson JA, Fox DM, Leshner AI, editors. Treating drug abusers effectively. New York: Blackwell; 1997. p. 253–79.
14. Huizinga D. Developmental sequences in delinquency: dynamic typologies. In: Crockett LJ, Crouter AC, editors. Pathways through adolescence. Mahwah (NJ): Lawrence Erlbaum; 1995. p. 15–34.
15. Loeber R, Keenan K, Zhang Q. Boys' experimentation and persistence in developmental pathways toward serious delinquency. J Child Fam Stud 1997;6:321–57.

16. Schoenwald SK, Rowland MD. Multisystemic therapy. In: Burns BJ, Hoagwood K, editors. Community treatment for youth: evidence-based interventions for severe emotional and behavioral disorders. New York: Oxford University Press; 2002. p. 91–116.

17. van Wijk A, Loeber R, Vermeiren R, et al. Violent juvenile sex offenders compared with violent juvenile nonsex offenders: explorative findings from the Pittsburgh Youth Study. Sex Abuse 2005;17:333–52.

18. Seto MC, Lalumière ML. What is so special about male adolescent sexual offending? A review and test of explanations through meta-analysis. Psychol Bull 2010; 136:526–75.

19. Saleh FM, Vincent GM. Juveniles who commit sex crimes. Adolesc Psychiatry 2004;28:183–207.

20. Cantor JM, Kuban ME, Blak T, et al. Physical height in pedophilic and hebephilic sexual offenders. Sex Abuse 2007;19:395–408.

21. Lane S. Assessment of sexually abusive youth. In: Ryan G, Lane S, editors. Juvenile sexual offending causes, consequences, and correction. San Francisco (CA): Jossey-Bass; 1997. p. 219–63.

22. Letourneau EJ. Guilt-phase testimony. The Forum 2003;15(3).

23. Association for the Treatment of Sexual Abusers. Practice standards and guidelines for members of the Association for the Treatment of Sexual Abusers. Beaverton (OR): Association for the Treatment of Sexual Abusers; 2005.

24. Worling JR. Adolescent sexual offender treatment at the SAFE-T program. In: Marshall WL, Fernandez YM, Hudson SM, et al, editors. Sourcebook of treatment programs for sexual offenders. New York: Plenum Press; 1998. p. 353–66.

25. Saunders EB, Awad GA. Assessment, management, and treatment planning for male adolescent sexual offenders. Am J Orthopsychiatry 1988;58(4):571–9.

26. Rich P. Understanding, assessing, and rehabilitating juvenile sexual offenders. Hoboken (NJ): John Wiley; 2003.

27. O'Reilly G, Carr A. The clinical assessment of young people with sexually abusive behaviour. In: O'Reilly G, Marshall WL, Carr A, et al, editors. The handbook of clinical intervention with young people who sexually abuse. New York: Brunner-Routledge; 2004. p. 163–90.

28. Achenbach TM. Youth self-report. Burlington (VT): University of Vermont, Research Center for Children, Youth, and Families; 1995.

29. Achenbach TM. Child behavior checklist for ages 6 to 18. Burlington (VT): University of Vermont, Research Center for Children, Youth, and Families; 2001.

30. Rescorla LA, Achenbach TM. The Achenbach system of empirically based assessment (ASEBA) for ages 18 to 90 years. Instruments for adults. In: Maruish ME, editor. The use of psychological testing for treatment planning and outcomes assessment, vol. 3. 3rd edition. Mahwah (NJ): Lawrence Erlbaum; 2004. p. 115–52.

31. Elliott DS, Huizinga D, Ageton SS. Explaining delinquency and drug use. Beverly Hills (CA): Sage; 1985.

32. Thornberry TP, Krohn MD. The self-report method for measuring delinquency and crime. Crim Justice 2000;4:33–83.

33. Becker JV, Kaplan MS. The assessment of adolescent sexual offenders. In: Prinz RJ, editor. Advances in behavioral assessment of children and families. Greenwich (CT): JAI Press; 1988. p. 97–118.

34. Hunter JA, Becker JV, Kaplan MS. The Adolescent Sexual Interest Card Sort: test-retest reliability and concurrent validity in relation to phallometric assessment. Arch Sex Behav 1995;24:555–61.

35. Nichols HR, Molinder I. Multiphasic sex inventory ii – adolescent male version. 2010. Available at: http://www.nicholsandmolinder.com/sex-offender-assessment-msi-ii-jm.php. Accessed April 13, 2011.

36. Friedrich WN, Lysne M, Sim L, et al. Assessing sexual behavior in high-risk adolescents with the Adolescent Clinical Sexual Behavior Inventory (ACSBI). Child Maltreat 2004;9(3):239–50.

37. Wherry JN, Berres AK, Sim L, et al. Factor structure of the Adolescent Clinical Sexual Behavior Inventory. J Child Sex Abus 2009;18(3):233–46.

38. Briere JN. Child abuse trauma: theory and treatment of the lasting effects. Newbury Park (CA): Sage; 1992.

39. Wolfe VV, Gentile C, Michienzi T, et al. The Children's Impact of Traumatic Events Scale: a measure of post-sexual abuse PTSD symptoms. Behav Assess 1991;13: 359–83.

40. Fischer L, Smith G. Statistical adequacy of the Abel Assessment for Interest in Paraphilias. Sex Abuse 1999;11(3):195–205.

41. Abel GG, Jordan A, Rouleau JL, et al. Use of visual reaction time to assess male adolescents who molest children. Sex Abuse 2004;16(3):255–65.

42. Worling J. Assessing sexual arousal with adolescent males who have offended sexually: self-report and unobtrusively measured viewing time. Sex Abuse 2006;18(4):383–400.

43. Fanniff AM, Becker JV. Specialized assessment and treatment of adolescent sex offenders. Aggression and Violent Behavior 2006;11:265–82.

44. Marshall WL, Fernandez YM. Phallometric testing with sexual offenders: theory, research, and practice. Brandon (VT): Safer Society Press; 2003.

45. Coric V, Feuerstein S, Fortunati F, et al. Assessing sex offenders. Psychiatry 2005; 2(11):26–9.

46. Henggeler SW, Schoenwald SK, Borduin CM, et al. Multisystemic treatment of antisocial behavior in children and adolescents. 2nd edition. New York: Guilford Press; 2009.

47. Clift RJ, Rajlic G, Gretton HM. Discriminative and predictive validity of penile plethysmograph in adolescent sex offenders. Sex Abuse 2009;21:335–62.

48. Seto MC, Lalumiere ML, Blanchard R. The discriminate validity of a phallometric test for pedophilic interests among adolescent sex offenders against children. Psychol Assess 2000;12(3):319–27.

49. Hindman J, Peters JM. Polygraph testing leads to better understanding adult and juvenile sex offenders. Fed Probat 2001;l65:8–15.

50. Grubin D, Madsen L, Parsons S, et al. A prospective study of the impact of the polygraphy on high risk behaviours in adult sex offenders. Sex Abuse 2004;16:209–22.

51. Emerick RL, Dutton WA. The effect of polygraphy on the self report of adolescent sex offenders: implications for risk assessment. Sex Abuse 1993;6:83–103.

52. National Research Council of the National Academies. The polygraph and lie detection. Washington, DC: The National Academies Press; 2003.

53. Rajlic G, Gretton HM. An examination of two sexual recidivism risk measures in adolescent offenders. Crim Justice Behav 2010;37:1066–85.

54. Viljoen JL, Elkovitch N, Scalora MJ, et al. Assessment of reoffense risk in adolescents who have committed sexual offenses: predictive validity of the ERASOR, PCL: YV, YLS/CMI, and Static-99. Crim Justice Behav 2009;36:981–1000.

55. Worling JR, Curwen T. Adolescent sexual offender recidivism: success of specialized treatment and implications for risk prediction. Child Abuse Negl 2001;24:965–82.

56. Prentky RA, Nien-Chen L, Righthand S, et al. Assessing risk of sexually abusive behavior among youth in a child welfare sample. Behav Sci Law 2010;28:24–45.

57. Worling JR. The Estimate of Risk of Adolescent Sexual Offense Recidivism (ERASOR): preliminary psychometric data. Sex Abuse 2004;16:235–54.
58. Viljoen JL, Scalora M, Cuadra L, et al. Assessing risk for violence in adolescents who have sexually offended a comparison of the J-SOAP-II, J-SORRAT-II, and SAVRY. Crim Justice Behav 2008;35:5–23.
59. Martinez R, Flores J, Rosenfeld B. Validity of the Juvenile Sex Offender Assessment Protocol–II (J-SOAP-II) in a sample of urban minority youth. Crim Justice Behav 2007;34:1284–95.
60. Parks GA, Bard DE. Risk factors for adolescent sex offender recidivism: evaluation of predictive factors and comparison of three groups based upon victim type. Sex Abuse 2006;18:319–42.
61. Caldwell M, Ziemke M, Vitacco M. An examination of the Sex Offender Registration and Notification Act as applied to juveniles: evaluating the ability to predict sexual recidivism. Psychol Public Pol L 2008;14:89–114.
62. Letourneau EJ, Armstrong KS. Recidivism rates for registered and nonregistered juvenile sexual offenders. Sex Abuse 2008;20:393–408.
63. Letourneau EJ, Bandyopadhyay D, Sinha D, et al. The influence of sex offender registration on juvenile sexual recidivism. Crim Justice Policy Rev 2009;20:136–53.
64. McGrath RJ, Cumming GF, Burchard BL. Current practices and trends in sexual abuser management: the Safer Society 2002 nationwide survey. Brandon (VT): Safer Society Press; 2003.
65. Worling JR, Litteljohn A, Bookalam D. 20-year prospective follow-up study of specialized treatment for adolescents who offended sexually. Behav Sci Law 2010;28:46–57.
66. Henggeler SW, Schoenwald SK, Borduin CM, et al. Multisystemic treatment of antisocial behavior in children and adolescents. New York: Guilford Press; 1998.
67. Schoenwald SK, Henggeler SW, Brondino MJ, et al. Multisystemic therapy: monitoring treatment fidelity. Fam Process 2000;39:83–103.
68. Letourneau EJ, Borduin CM, Schaeffer CM. Multisystemic therapy for youth with problem sexual behaviors. In: Beech A, Craig L, Browne K, editors. Assessment and treatment of sexual offenders: a handbook. London: John Wiley; 2008. p. 453–72.
69. Henggeler SW, Letourneau EJ, Chapman JE, et al. Mediators of change for multisystemic therapy with juvenile sexual offenders. J Consult Clin Psychol 2009;77: 451–62.
70. Borduin CM, Henggeler SW, Blaske DM, et al. Multisystemic treatment of adolescent sexual offenders. Int J Offender Ther Comp Criminol 1990;35:105–14.
71. Borduin CM, Schaeffer CM. Multisystemic treatment of juvenile sexual offenders: a progress report. J Psychol Human Sex 2001;13:25–42.
72. Hollis S, Campbell F. What is meant by intention to treat analysis? Survey of published randomized controlled trials. BMJ 1999;319:670–4.
73. Hanson RK, Gordon A, Harris AJ, et al. First report of the Collaborative Outcomes Data Project on the effectiveness of psychological treatment for sex offenders. Sex Abuse 2002;14:169–94.
74. Carpentier M, Silovsky JF, Chaffin M. Randomized trial of treatment for children with sexual behavior problems: ten-year follow-up. J Consult Clin Psychol 2006; 74:482–8.
75. Chaffin M, Berliner L, Block R, et al. Report of the ATSA task force on children with sexual behavior problems. Child Maltreat 2008;13:199–218.
76. DiIulio JJ Jr. How to stop the coming crime wave. New York: Manhattan Institute; 1996.
77. Roper, Superintendent, Potosi Correctional Center v Simmons, 543 U.S. 551 (2005).

The Supreme Court and the Sentencing of Juveniles in the United States: Reaffirming the Distinctiveness of Youth

David M. Siegel, JD

KEYWORDS

- Sentencing • Juveniles • Imprisonment • Proportionality
- Developmental

During the late 1960s and 1970s, the US Supreme Court applied most of the basic procedural guarantees in adult criminal cases to juveniles, thereby constitutionally defining the contemporary juvenile justice process. In less than a decade, the Court held that juveniles charged with delinquent offenses (what would be crimes were they adults) had the right to be represented by counsel and receive notice of the charges, as well as the trial rights of the privilege against compelled self-incrimination and the right to confrontation and cross-examination.[1] The Court recognized that delinquent offenses required proof beyond a reasonable doubt,[2] and the prohibition against double jeopardy also applied in delinquency proceedings.[3] Although every procedure in a juvenile delinquency proceeding did not have to be identical to that in an adult criminal trial (juries were held not to be required in delinquency adjudications[4]), even less comprehensive proceedings than a juvenile adjudication, transfers to criminal court, now demanded a degree of procedural regularity and formality previously unknown in juvenile court.[5]

After that period, the Court stayed out of regulating the juvenile system, even throughout the dramatic increase in its punitive aspects during the 1980s and 1990s. It upheld the constitutionality of the juvenile death penalty in 4 homicide cases

Financial disclosure and conflicts of interest: the author has nothing to disclose.

New England Law | Boston, Center for Law and Social Responsibility, 154 Stuart Street, Boston, MA 02116, USA

E-mail address: dsiegel@nesl.edu

Child Adolesc Psychiatric Clin N Am 20 (2011) 431–445

doi:10.1016/j.chc.2011.03.011

childpsych.theclinics.com

1056-4993/11/$ – see front matter © 2011 Elsevier Inc. All rights reserved.

during the 1980s and never definitively set a minimum age for its application.[6–8] The Court recognized that youth could be a mitigating factor that required consideration in capital sentencing, but refused in 1982 to hold the death penalty categorically inapplicable to 16-year-olds.[6] In 1988, 4 Justices found it categorically inapplicable to 15-year-olds (as cruel and unusual punishment given an evolving national consensus)[7] and noted an accepted presentation concerning a psychological study of 14 juveniles sentenced to death[9] had found that beyond the "maturational stresses [of adolescence], homicidal adolescents must cope with brain dysfunction, cognitive limitations, and severe psychopathology."[7] However, in the next term, 5 justices rejected the argument that capital punishment was categorically inapplicable to 16-year-olds and 17-year-olds, finding no national consensus on the juvenile death penalty.[8]

This approach changed in the first decade of the twenty-first century, because the Court twice set key limits on severe juvenile sentences, invalidating the juvenile death penalty in *Roper v Simmons*[10] and juvenile sentences of life without possibility of parole (LWOP) for nonhomicide offenses in *Graham v Florida*.[11] Unlike jurisprudential developments of the 1960s and 1970s, which simply applied to juveniles the greater procedural protection the Court was generally affording adult criminal defendants, there has been no corresponding sentencing relaxation for adults to accompany the more recent juvenile decisions. Instead, *Roper* and *Graham* forthrightly hold that juveniles' distinctive characteristics require different legal treatment than that permitted adults in the criminal justice system. This rationale conflicts with legal developments across individual states since the 1980s that have subjected younger children to harsher sentences for more offenses as juvenile offenders and that have increased the range of children and offenses susceptible to transfer for trial as adults. The Court's new reasoning is instead a genuine developmental approach to juvenile justice, which may therefore also undermine other juvenile sentencing practices, such as very long sentences for nonhomicides that are effectively LWOP, sentences of LWOP for homicides, very young ages for transfer for trial as an adult, and perhaps even very young susceptibility to juvenile adjudication.

TWENTY-FIRST CENTURY APPROACH TO JUVENILE SENTENCING

The Court's recognition, in categorical challenges to certain juvenile sentences, of distinctive psychological and cognitive features of juveniles that render them less culpable and afford them greater rehabilitative potential than adult offenders, applies well beyond the categories (the death penalty and LWOP for nonhomicides) in which the Court has considered them in *Roper* and *Graham*. The proportionality framework for categorical challenges to sentencing as cruel and unusual punishment and these key decisions are discussed later. This article also suggests how the reasoning underlying these cases might affect juvenile sentencing, and juvenile justice, in the future.

One important legal caveat about these 2 decisions could affect their future impact: both were closely divided opinions, in which the core rationale that juveniles' distinctive features make them less culpable than adults who commit the same offenses obtained the slimmest possible majority of 5 votes. (Both majority opinions were authored by Justice Anthony Kennedy.) The closeness of the votes does not undermine the decisions' precedential value but does suggest how easily the jurisprudence might change when the Court's composition changes, especially because the Court accepted a categorical challenge to these sentences based heavily on its own assessment of proportionality.

CATEGORICAL LIMITS ON SENTENCING LESS THAN THE EIGHTH AMENDMENT

The Eighth Amendment to the US Constitution's prohibition against cruel and unusual punishment[12] ("Excessive bail shall not be required, nor excessive fines imposed, nor cruel and unusual punishments inflicted."), applicable to the states through the Fourteenth Amendment, imposes some degree of proportionality between punishment and crime, but the definitions of, and penalties for, crimes are largely committed to the states. A penalty can be cruel and unusual as applied to a specific offender in a specific case, but, given states' latitude in setting crimes and penalties, and the infinite variety of facts in every case and circumstances of every offender, the Court since 1991 has required gross disproportionality between crime and punishment before it will even examine a particular punishment in a specific case.[13] (It will then compare a particular defendant's sentence with others imposed for similar crimes in the state or for the same crimes in other states.)[13] Thus, it has upheld extremely long sentences (including LWOP) for nonhomicides and even for nonviolent offenses, such as possession of more than 650 g of cocaine with intent to distribute,[13] as well as harsh sentencing schemes such as so-called 3-strikes provisions, applied to impose 2 consecutive sentences of 25 years to life for a third, nonviolent, felony conviction.[14] Although 2 state supreme courts had found LWOP sentences for 2 specific juveniles disproportionate (1 for a homicide[15] and 1 for a nonhomicide[16]) many had upheld such LWOP sentences against claims that, as applied, they were disproportionate,[17,18] even for children as young as 12 years of age.[19]

Unlike as-applied proportionality analysis, in a facial or categorical challenge, the Court examines whether a given penalty imposed for a certain crime is disproportionate for an entire class of offenders, on its face, regardless of the facts and circumstances in any case. This categorical review of proportionality involves 2 steps: first, an assessment of the "evolving standards of decency that mark the progress of a maturing society"[20] to determine whether there are objective indicia of a national consensus against a particular penalty, and, second, the Court's own assessment, based on its jurisprudence, the amendment's text, history, meaning and purpose, whether the punishment is disproportionate. Although the Court has invalidated a few noncapital penalties as categorically cruel and unusual,[20–22] in the last half-century, virtually all such decisions have involved the death penalty.[23–25]

The "clearest and most reliable objective evidence of contemporary values is the legislation enacted by the country's legislatures."[26] Typically, the Court has interpreted this to mean how many states' laws permit a particular penalty, because states prohibiting a penalty have arguably found it cruel or at least disproportionate. It has also assessed the frequency with which a certain permissible penalty is imposed, on the theory that a penalty imposed very infrequently is unusual. There is no specific quantitative test for a national consensus, and the Court has considered not only prohibition of penalties but also legal trends in changes to available penalties.

THE DEATH PENALTY: ROPER V SIMMONS (2005)

Christopher Simmons was 17 years old when he organized a residential burglary and murder with 2 other juveniles. As the instigator, he described in chilling, callous terms the plan to break in, bind and remove the female resident, and throw her off a bridge to drown, "assur[ing] his friends they could 'get away with it' because they were minors."[10] Simmons and 1 juvenile (the other dropped out) went through with the plan, and Simmons' later accounts confirmed that he knew the victim from a prior auto accident with her and that he had killed her so she could not identify him.[10] Although expert testimony at later postconviction proceedings emphasized

Simmons's impulsiveness, lack of maturity, and susceptibility to being manipulated or influenced, the facts of his own crime did not suggest these qualities. When the Court accepted Simmons' case, instead of assessing whether the death penalty was cruel and unusual as applied to him, the Court considered whether imposition of capital punishment on an entire category of offenders (persons who are juveniles at the time of their offense) was cruel and unusual.

The US Supreme Court has examined mental retardation and youth, both mitigating factors in capital sentencing, in claims that the death penalty was categorically cruel and unusual punishment. It had considered and rejected both, in unrelated cases decided the same day in 1989,[8,27] but in 2002 the Court reexamined mental retardation and recognized in *Atkins v Virginia* an evolving national consensus that the death penalty was categorically inappropriate for retarded offenders.[26] It also found that mentally retarded defendants were less culpable, given the lack of deterrence and retributive effect punishment could have on them because of their distinctive limitations as opposed to other defendants, which also reduced their ability to interact with the legal system as defendants, thereby subjecting them to a higher risk of wrongful conviction.[26]

Drawing on *Atkins*, the Missouri Supreme Court had ruled that, even though Simmons had received a fair trial and an effective defense, imposing the death penalty on him, as a juvenile, was categorically cruel and unusual punishment for the same reasons that it was cruel and unusual to apply it to mentally retarded defendants: because juveniles were less culpable than adults, less able to deliberate about their actions, and thus less likely to be meaningfully deterred by the prospect of punishment. Although presented with "numerous current studies and scientific articles about the structure of the human mind, the continuing growth of those portions of the mind that control maturity and decision-making during adolescence and young adulthood, and the lesser ability of teenagers to reason," the Missouri Supreme Court found that it did not need to rely on these.[28]

When Simmons' case reached the US Supreme Court, it too directly applied its analysis in *Atkins*, but, unlike the Missouri Supreme Court, it did explicitly address, and accept, the developmental and psychological distinctiveness of adolescents.[10] (Both the American Psychological Association[29] and the American Psychiatric Association, the latter in conjunction with the American Medical Association, filed amicus curiae briefs supporting Simmons.[30]) The Court first recognized a national consensus against the imposition of the juvenile death penalty, based on 30 of the 50 states that did not allow it, although this included (as had its calculus of the national consensus on imposition of the death penalty on the mentally retarded) the 12 states that then prohibited all capital punishment. It then conducted its own proportionality analysis, focused (because the death penalty is the most severe penalty) on whether it was "limited to those offenders who commit 'a narrow category of the most serious crimes' and whose extreme culpability makes them 'the most deserving of execution.'"[10]

The Court then identified 3 features of juveniles' distinctiveness that interfered with the operation of the criminal justice system on them and which therefore prevented their reliable classification as the most culpable offenders. The Court acknowledged 3 distinctive features of adolescence: immaturity that leads to reckless behavior, susceptibility to negative and outside influences, especially peer pressure, and more transitory personality traits than those of adults.[10] It is this recognition in *Simmons* of categorical distinctiveness that gives the decision significance beyond capital punishment, because these features of adolescence potentially apply to all delinquent juveniles.

None of these propositions were novel when the Court recognized them in 2005, but the Court did acknowledge scientific as well as legal (and experiential) sources for them, although often not the most recent of such sources. The Court noted the recognized immaturity of adolescents, often accompanied by reckless conduct (citing the 1992 statement by Jeffrey Arnett, presented in the brief of the American Psychological Association: "[I]t has been noted that 'adolescents are overrepresented statistically in virtually every category of reckless behavior'"[31]), reflected in many legal restrictions on juveniles engaging in otherwise lawful conduct such as voting, jury service, and marriage. Concerning juveniles' susceptibility to outside influences, the Court noted the unassailably correct fact that children, as legally controlled by others, have less ability to remove themselves from deleterious situations than do adults, citing a statement by Laurence Steinberg and Elizabeth Scott, from an article cited in both the American Psychological Association's amicus brief and the amicus brief of the American Psychiatric Association and American Medical Association, that "as legal minors, [juveniles] lack the freedom that adults have to extricate themselves from a criminogenic setting."[32] For the transitory nature of adolescent personality traits, for example, the Court cited Erik Erikson's 1968 *Identity: Youth and Crisis*.

These differences mean that juveniles are less morally responsible for criminal conduct than would be an adult:

> The susceptibility of juveniles to immature and irresponsible behavior means "their irresponsible conduct is not as morally reprehensible as that of an adult." Their own vulnerability and comparative lack of control over their immediate surroundings mean juveniles have a greater claim than adults to be forgiven for failing to escape negative influences in their whole environment. The reality that juveniles still struggle to define their identity means it is less supportable to conclude that even a heinous crime committed by a juvenile is evidence of irretrievably depraved character. From a moral standpoint it would be misguided to equate the failings of a minor with those of an adult, for a greater possibility exists that a minor's character deficiencies will be reformed. Indeed, "[t]he relevance of youth as a mitigating factor derives from the fact that the signature qualities of youth are transient; as individuals mature, the impetuousness and recklessness that may dominate in younger years can subside."[10] (Citations omitted.)

One other observation by the Court is noteworthy, because it relies on psychiatric diagnosis for the conclusion that juveniles are less culpable than adults. The Court pointed out that the difficulty of determining the cause of juveniles' behavior, which led the *Diagnostic and Statistical Manual of Mental Disorders*, Fourth Edition, to preclude a diagnosis of antisocial personality disorder until age 18 years, surely should give pause before jurors are asked to make a similar determination in capital sentencing.[10]

LIFE WITHOUT PAROLE FOR NONHOMICIDE OFFENSES: GRAHAM V FLORIDA (2010)

The US Supreme Court's most recent assessment of juvenile sentencing, *Graham v Florida*,[11] relied on its 2005 findings in *Roper* that juveniles had reduced culpability because of "lack of maturity and underdeveloped sense of responsibility," greater "vulnerab[ility] or susceptib[ility] to negative influence and outside pressure, including peer pressure," and that "their characters are not as well formed."[11] In *Roper*, the Court used these findings to conclude that reduced culpability implied correspondingly reduced punishment to invalidate the death penalty for offenses committed by juveniles. In *Graham*, it used these findings to invalidate a sentence of LWOP for a nonhomicide offense, holding that such juveniles sentenced to life must have "some realistic opportunity to obtain release before the end of that term."[11] Graham's case itself graphically shows both the legal susceptibility juveniles face to much harsher punishment and the basis for the clinical skepticism about juvenile decision making.

Terrance Jamar Graham, born to cocaine-addicted parents, was diagnosed with attention-deficit/hyperactivity disorder in grade school. He was drinking alcohol and smoking tobacco by age 9 years and using marijuana by 13 years. At age 16 years, with a ninth grade education and no prior juvenile adjudications or criminal convictions,[33] he attempted to rob a restaurant with 3 other juveniles. One juvenile, an employee, left the back door unlocked, through which Graham and 2 codefendants entered at closing time wearing masks. An accomplice struck the manager on his head with a metal bar (the manager required stitches) and all 3 fled without taking any money.[11]

Exercising his discretion to prosecute Graham directly as an adult, the prosecutor charged him with armed burglary with assault and attempted armed robbery. The burglary, a first-degree felony, carried a maximum possible sentence of LWOP; the attempted robbery carried a maximum sentence of 15 years' imprisonment. Graham had no prior juvenile record and, on his guilty plea, the Court deferred adjudication and imposed 2 concurrent 3-year terms of probation, all of which were suspended except for 12 months in jail. Barely 5 months after his release, Graham and 2 adults allegedly forced their way into a house, held the residents at gunpoint and ransacked the home.[11] In an alleged second robbery attempt that evening, a cohort of Graham's was shot and Graham, driving his family's car, dropped the others at a hospital. When police tried to stop him, he led them on a high-speed chase that ended in a crash. Three handguns were found in his car on his arrest.[11]

Graham denied involvement in the crimes, but when asked how many more robberies he had been involved in before that night, he said "2 to 3 before tonight." Graham was charged not with these crimes but with violating probation from his earlier offenses and, at a subsequent probation violation hearing, Graham admitted fleeing from the police (in violation of probation). The court found he had also violated probation by possessing weapons, associating with those engaged in crime, and committing a home-invasion robbery.

Graham was then sentenced for the first offense he had committed (for which he had been on probation). Facing a minimum of 5 years imprisonment and a maximum of LWOP, the defense sought 5 years and the prosecution recommended 30 years on the attempted burglary and 15 on the attempted robbery. The judge sentenced Graham to LWOP.

Several aspects of Graham's conduct and his interaction with the legal system exemplify the clinical conclusions about adolescent understanding and behavior and the consequences of the law's increasingly punitive approach to juveniles. From a legal perspective, it shows the extraordinary discretion committed to prosecutors, the ease of transfer for trial as adults, and the dramatically punitive consequences of the sentencing schemes to which juveniles were now susceptible. (The Court also noted this: "Many states have chosen to move away from juvenile court systems and to allow juveniles to be transferred to, or charged directly in, adult court under certain circumstances."[11]) Graham's first case could have been handled as a juvenile or adult offense; the discretion to directly file adult charges against someone aged 16 or 17 years old for certain felonies punishable by life or death was given to Florida prosecutors in 1978.[34] Before that, prosecutors had to file a motion in juvenile court for waiver of jurisdiction to adult criminal court. The decision to charge Graham as an adult was now solely the prosecutor's and it was not subject to review. The exposure to a lengthy sentence as an adult made a guilty plea to a sentence involving a comparatively short initial period of incarceration (1 year) followed by probation highly attractive, but these same severe potential consequences also made him eligible, for a single incident of violent crime at age 16 years, to a sentence of LWOP for violating probation. Graham's entire incarceration history before his sentence of LWOP was 1 year (at age 16 years) in a local jail.

Graham's case also reflects characteristic adolescent decision making that may be particularly relevant in culpability determinations. Although late adolescents may have the cognitive capacity to understand and reason as adults,[35] in practice judgments are highly affected by psychosocial factors that influence our values and preferences. Developmental psychologists have identified 4 ways psychosocial influences can increase adolescents' likelihood of criminal behavior: peer influence, adolescents' perspective on time, adolescents' perspective on risk, and their preference for risk. Peer influence, through social comparison and conformity, makes adolescents more likely to conform their behavior to that of others and measure their own behavior against that of others.[35] Graham's first case involved 3 juvenile codefendants, 1 of whom possessed and used a weapon. His second case (the probation violation), involved 2 adult accomplices who were 3 years older than him. Risk perception among adolescents also differs from that of adults, inclining them to undertake riskier behavior, and they also seem less risk averse than adults. Graham's early use of alcohol, tobacco, and drugs, as well as his readiness to engage in criminal conduct soon after release on probation, might fit these characteristics. In addition, adolescents have a different understanding of time, discounting the future more than adults. Two aspects of Graham's case show this. First, when he initially pled guilty, he asked for a second chance and promised to "do whatever it takes to get to the NFL." Second, his readiness to engage in conduct that would violate his probation and subject him to imprisonment for LWOP seems almost incomprehensible. It certainly seemed incomprehensible to the sentencing judge, which shows the legal system's lack of recognition of adolescent decision-making tendencies:

Mr Graham, as I look back on your case, yours is really candidly a sad situation. You had, as far as I can tell, you have quite a family structure. You had a lot of people who wanted to try and help you get your life turned around including the court system, and you had a judge who took the step to try and give you direction through his probation order to give you a chance to get back onto track. And at the time you seemed through your letters that that is exactly what you wanted to do. And I don't know why it is that you threw your life away. I don't know why.

But you did, and that is what is so sad about this today is that you have actually been given a chance to get through this, the original charge, which were very serious charges to begin with .... The attempted robbery with a weapon was a very serious charge.

And I don't understand why you would be given such a great opportunity to do something with your life and why you would throw it away. The only thing that I can rationalize is that you decided that this is how you were going to lead your life and that there is nothing that we can do for you. And as the State pointed out, that this is an escalating pattern of criminal conduct on your part and that we can't help you any further. We can't do anything to deter you. This is the way you are going to lead your life, and I don't know why you are going to. You've made that decision. I have no idea. But, evidently, that is what you decided to do.

I have reviewed the statute. I don't see where any further juvenile sanctions would be appropriate. I don't see where any youthful offender sanctions would be appropriate. Given your escalating pattern of criminal conduct, it is apparent to the Court that you have decided that this is the way you are going to live your life and that the only thing I can do now is to try and protect the community from your actions.[11]

The Court held in *Graham* that a sentence of LWOP for a juvenile was disproportionate for a nonhomicide offense, and as disproportionate it was cruel and unusual punishment in violation of the Eighth Amendment. Although the Court could have analyzed Graham's case solely as a claim that his sentence in his case was disproportionate to his crime (ie, as applied), it instead treated it as a categorical or facial challenge to the type of punishment (LWOP) for a class of defendants (juveniles charged with nonhomicide offenses) as a whole. Graham's was the first modern non–death penalty case in which the Court had used the categorical approach.

As for the evolving national consensus concerning LWOP for juveniles, although most states (37) plus the District of Columbia and federal law permitted sentences of LWOP for juvenile nonhomicide offenses, the Court found this of little importance because the sentence was imposed in only 12 of these jurisdictions for a total of 129 juveniles serving sentences of LWOP for nonhomicide offenses, more than half of whom (77) were in Florida.[11] The Court acknowledged several shortcomings in its assessment of a national consensus: it could not, with precision, identify all juveniles who had been sentenced to LWOP for nonhomicide offenses, or the total number of juveniles who could have been sentenced to LWOP. The absolute number of LWOP sentences imposed on juveniles for nonhomicides was still far greater than other sentencing practices the Court had invalidated and, even excluding states that had imposed LWOP for juvenile nonhomicides, still more than half of all states (26) did not specifically bar the practice. However, the Court concluded that the "many States that allow life without parole for juvenile non-homicide offenses but do not impose the punishment should not be treated as if they have expressed the view that the sentence is appropriate. The sentencing practice now under consideration is exceedingly rare."[11]

The critical portion of the Court's analysis thus was its own judgment about the appropriateness of the penalty given the culpability of the offenders. Here, it began with its conclusion in *Roper* that "as compared with adults, juveniles have a 'lack of maturity and an underdeveloped sense of responsibility'; they 'are more vulnerable or susceptible to negative influences and outside pressures, including peer pressure,' and their characters are 'not as well formed'."[11] These characteristics, which the Court had held in *Roper*, made it difficult even for experts to distinguish between transient immaturity and irreparable corruption (preventing the death penalty from reliably being applied to the worst offenders) were even better established in 2010 than they had been when the Court considered the juvenile death penalty in 2005.[11] Citing amicus briefs filed by the American Psychological Association and on behalf of both the American Medical and American Psychiatric Associations, "Developments in psychology and brain science continue to show fundamental differences between juvenile and adult minds."[11] These characteristics meant juveniles have greater potential for change, thus it is both harder to conclude why the juvenile acted as he did and there is greater potential for rehabilitation.

The Court specifically did not hold that juveniles sentenced to life were entitled to release at a specific point or a sentence of a specific term of years; it held that they are entitled to "some meaningful opportunity to obtain release based on demonstrated maturity and rehabilitation."[11] The Court then rejected case-by-case (ie, as applied) determination of proportionality on bases that may suggest future challenges to aspects of the juvenile justice system more generally. Florida argued that, because Graham's prosecution as an adult had been an exercise of prosecutorial discretion, then age was being taken into account as a sentencing factor, and so, even if Graham's sentence was excessive in his case, age could in future cases continue to be taken into account on a case-by-case basis without invalidating the penalty categorically.

The Court rejected this argument for 3 reasons. First, for the same reason it had rejected in *Roper* case-by-case application of the juvenile death penalty: the fundamental differences between juveniles and adults made it too difficult to accurately assess culpability and the Court found that even if LWOP was somehow appropriate for the most heinous offenses, "It does not follow that courts taking a case-by-case proportionality approach could with sufficient accuracy distinguish the few incorrigible juvenile offenders from the many that have the capacity for change."[11] Second, the Court noted, it ignores the systematic ways in which juveniles are less able to effectively be represented. The same cognitive features of adolescents' decision making that make them likely to become defendants (their inability to assess long-term consequences and their youthful rebelliousness) also make them particularly difficult defendants to represent, because they may make poor strategic decisions and have difficulty interacting with adult counsel.[11] Third, the Court made an existential argument: anything less than a categorical ban on LWOP would deprive some juveniles "of the opportunity to achieve maturity of judgment and self-recognition of human worth and potential."[11]

EVOLVING DEVELOPMENTAL CONCEPTION OF YOUTH

The reasoning in *Roper* and *Graham* establishes what might be termed developmental culpability: the concept that distinctive developmental psychosocial, psychological, cognitive, and neuroanatomic characteristics of youth make juveniles less culpable as a class than adults who commit the same offenses. However, much of the scientific research underlying this legal concept, some of which the Court cited, also supports concepts of developmental competence or developmental capacity, suggesting that juveniles lack certain cognitive and psychological abilities to meaningfully undergo the process of adjudication in the juvenile justice system. The concepts of developmental culpability explicitly embraced in *Roper* and *Graham*, and developmental competency or capacity, on which *Roper* and *Graham* are implicitly premised, suggest 2 different types of future challenges in juvenile cases.

The concept of developmental culpability suggests challenges to specific sentencing practices in juvenile cases related to those invalidated in *Roper* and *Graham*. Likely targets include sentences of LWOP for homicides committed by juveniles, especially those in which juveniles did not kill, intend to kill, or foresee death, and very long sentences that are terms of years for both homicides and nonhomicides committed by juveniles and challenges to broader trends in the juvenile justice system. The broader challenges to aspects of the juvenile justice system based on the reasoning in these cases possibly include transfer provisions allowing transfer of younger children, challenges to juveniles' competence to be adjudicated, and perhaps even resurrection of the infancy defense.

ROLE OF THE MENTAL HEALTH SCIENCES IN THE DEVELOPMENTAL CONCEPTION

The US Supreme Court's recognition of adolescents' psychological, cognitive, and neuroanatomic distinctiveness did not come by chance. In both *Roper* and *Graham*, amicus briefs were submitted by the American Psychiatric Association in conjunction with the American Medical Association (the APA-AMA Brief)[30,36] and the American Psychological Association (the APA Brief).[29,37] In *Roper*, both sets of briefs supported Simmons, arguing much the same propositions, although with slightly different emphasis. The APA-AMA argued that "older adolescents behave differently than adults because their minds operate differently, their emotions are more volatile, and their brains are anatomically immature'."[30] It argued that cognitive deficiencies in even older adolescents inherently made them risk takers. These deficiencies rendered adolescents less able to accurately conduct cost-benefit assessments, to overvalue gain, underestimate loss, and to overemphasize present, rather than future, consequences. The APA similarly explained, "Adolescent decision-makers on average are less future-oriented and less likely to consider properly the consequences of their actions."[29] These cognitive deficiencies were magnified by shortcomings in social and emotional capability, limiting adolescents' abilities to act independently, to view events from the perspectives of others, and to control impulsiveness. These cognitive deficiencies were also especially pronounced when other psychological or psychosocial factors came into play, including stress, emotions, and peer pressure.

These lessons from cognitive psychology were then supported with results of brain magnetic resonance imaging (MRI) and functional MRI (fMRI) studies, which had not existed when the Court considered the juvenile death penalty in the 1980s. Both briefs argued that 2 findings of this research were critical for assessment of adolescent culpability. First, that adolescents rely for certain tasks much more than adults on the amygdala, and, second, that the portions of the brain involving so-called executive function develop last, often after late adolescence. Both also detailed 2 specific anatomic processes that are measures of brain maturity, myelination and pruning, which showed considerable maturation during late adolescence and into adulthood, especially in the areas of the brain related to impulse-control, risk assessment, and moral reasoning.[29,30] In *Graham*, although all 3 organizations made similar points, the APA-AMA brief did not support either side, whereas the APA brief supported *Graham*. The Court cited both briefs for the proposition that its conclusions about the distinctive characteristics of juveniles in *Roper* were better established in 2010 than they had been in 2005.[11]

SPECIFIC CHALLENGES BASED ON DEVELOPMENTAL CULPABILITY
Sentences of LWOP for Homicide Offenses

Proportionality of punishment depends on the offense, the offender, and the amount of punishment. Sentences of LWOP for homicides committed by a juvenile involve the same offender and amount of punishment rejected in *Graham*, thus, if LWOP for homicides committed by juveniles is distinguishable, it must be because of the severity of the offense. A homicide is undoubtedly a more serious offense than a nonhomicide, and the Court has restricted the most severe punishment available to adults (the death penalty) to homicides, rejecting it for the rape of an adult woman[24] or a child[25] and homicides in which the offender himself did not kill (ie, a codefendant killed), did not intend to kill, or did not foresee that death would occur (ie, a felony murder, in which the homicide legally became a murder because it occurred during commission of a felony).[23]

After *Roper*, the justifications for punishment never merit the death penalty when the homicide is committed by a juvenile. After *Graham*, the justifications for punishment never merit LWOP when any nonhomicide is committed by a juvenile. Do the justifications for punishment that the Court has accepted as meriting either the death penalty or LWOP for homicides committed by adults merit LWOP when the homicide is committed by a juvenile?

Homicide sentences most likely to face proportionality challenges are juvenile murders in which the juvenile did not personally kill, intend to kill, or foresee that death would occur, because the Supreme Court has already barred the death penalty for these homicides when committed by adults.[23] If the most severe penalty available for adults is disproportionate for these offenses, is the most severe penalty available for juveniles (possibly LWOP for juvenile homicides) also disproportionate for these offenses? These categorical challenges are just beginning, and, so far, have been rejected by an appellate court for a 14-year-old codefendant convicted of fatally beating a robbery victim and then setting his trailer home on fire,[38] and by a trial court for a juvenile accomplice to a felony murder who did not cause the victim's death.[39]

Proportionality of punishment, apart from the defendant's characteristics, depends on the severity of the offense and the degree to which the punishment advances legitimate penological goals. A punishment is, by its nature, disproportionate if it has no legitimate penological justification.[11] Of the 4 justifications for punishment, the Court has recognized (retribution, deterrence, incapacitation, and rehabilitation), clearly LWOP does not advance rehabilitation. As the Court noted in *Graham*, LWOP, by definition, "foreswears altogether the rehabilitative ideal."[11] A sentence of LWOP advances incapacitation, although it does so by making a judgment of incorrigibility that the Court finds cannot be made of a juvenile. The majority's opinion in *Graham* provides both an opening to argue that LWOP for juvenile homicides is disproportionate (because incapacitation is based on an unreliable determination of incorrigibility) and carefully limited phrases with which to respond to these arguments ("[W]hile incapacitation may be a legitimate penological goal sufficient to justify life without parole in other contexts, it is inadequate to justify that punishment for juveniles *who did not commit homicide*"[11] [Emphasis added.]).

The goals of retribution or deterrence could present different analyses for a sentence of LWOP imposed for a homicide as opposed to a nonhomicide, although *Roper* suggests otherwise with respect to retribution. *Roper* established that, even in the case of a homicide, "whether viewed as an attempt to express the community's moral outrage or as an attempt to right the balance for the wrong to the victim, the case for retribution is not as strong with a minor as with an adult."[10] Deterrence seems an especially weak basis on which to premise an LWOP sentence for a juvenile, because of the decision-making weaknesses of adolescents identified by the Court in *Graham* and *Roper*.

Lengthy Sentence that is Effectively LWOP

Does a 100-year sentence provide "some meaningful opportunity to obtain release based on demonstrated maturity and rehabilitation"? If LWOP is disproportionate when applied to juveniles because of their characteristics, other sentences whose long periods before parole eligibility make them indistinguishable from LWOP are also arguably cruel and unusual because the relevant characteristics of the juvenile defendant are the same. These characteristics include the risk of error in sentencing because of the brutality or callousness of the crime (which might merit a 100-year sentence) that might lead a sentencer to overlook a "juvenile offender's objective immaturity, vulnerability and lack of true depravity"[11] and the special disadvantages juveniles have as criminal defendants because of their distinctive personality and cognitive features.

What does "some meaningful opportunity to obtain release based on demonstrated maturity and rehabilitation" mean? There is no constitutional requirement that states have a system of parole,[40] and, even in such a system, there is "no constitutional or inherent right of a convicted person to be conditionally released before the expiration of a valid sentence."[40] The Court's entire explanation was this:

It is for the State, in the first instance, to explore the means and mechanisms for compliance. It bears emphasis, however, that while the Eighth Amendment

*forbids a State from imposing a life without parole sentence on a juvenile nonho-
micide offender, it does not require the State to release that offender during his
natural life. Those who commit truly horrifying crimes as juveniles may turn out
to be irredeemable, and thus deserving of incarceration for the duration of their
lives. The Eighth Amendment does not foreclose the possibility that persons
convicted of nonhomicide crimes committed before adulthood will remain behind
bars for life. It does forbid States from making the judgment at the outset that
those offenders never will be fit to reenter society.[11]*

A sentence with parole eligibility so far in the future that a juvenile defendant might
not survive to reach it seems an equivalent effect; how much less of a sentence might
reach this level is unclear.

GENERAL CHALLENGES BASED ON DEVELOPMENTAL COMPETENCE OR CAPACITY
Transfer or Waiver to Adult Court

Although *Roper* and *Graham* involved constitutional challenges to punishment, the
underlying reasoning of these decisions (that juveniles are distinct from adults in
ways that make treating them the same cruel and unusual punishment) could be applicable to other aspects of the juvenile justice system, not as a challenge to punishment
but possibly as one based on either the Equal Protection or Due Process clauses of
the Fourteenth Amendment.

In December 2005, the American Psychiatric Association adopted a Position Statement, *Adjudication of Youths as Adults in the Criminal Justice System*, which specifically encouraged a developmental approach to juvenile justice and urged reform of the
use of transfer or waiver to adult court. It specifically recommended:

*(1) a moratorium on the expansion of eligibility criteria for transfer; (2) limiting
transfer only to judicial discretion (or sole authority by judge); (3) an elimination
of transfers for non-violent offenders; (4) an elimination of transfer of first-time
offenders; [and] (5) the development of specialized facilities for transferred
youth.[41]*

Competence or Capacity

Both *Roper* and *Graham* recognize distinctive developmental features of juveniles
and young adults that distinguish them from adults and make them, as a group,
less culpable than adults. Punishment theorists have argued that the legal age of
majority or lawful conduct in areas other than criminal law suggests that juveniles
are systematically less able to participate meaningfully in the justice system as criminal defendants. Developmental psychologists have been studying the abilities of
juveniles relevant to being a criminal defendant for several decades.[42] There is
a 4-part framework first set forth by Bonnie[43] for evaluating abilities relevant to an
individual's being a criminal defendant: abilities to (1) understand the legal process,
(2) appreciate the significance of legal circumstances for one's own situation, (3)
communicate information, and (4) use reasoning and judgment in decisions.
Grisso[42] used this framework to report in a summary of research on these questions
in 2000 that "compared with adults, youths under age fifteen are at greater risk of
having a poor knowledge of matters related to their participation in trials. For
adolescents fifteen and older, on average their understanding may be more like
that of adults."

The MacArthur Foundation's Research Network on Adolescent Development and
Juvenile Justice has been collecting data on issues related to juvenile capacity for

more than a decade, and has presented its results in a series of papers and issue briefs.[44] Network researchers interviewed 1400 individuals, aged 11 to 24 years, in juvenile detention facilities and the community, to compare the abilities of teens versus young adults regarding competence to stand trial. "Those aged 11–13 performed significantly worse than 14–15 year olds, who performed significantly worse than 16–17 year olds and 18–24 year olds (adults)."[45] Researchers also found that emotional maturity levels dramatically affected legal decision making of teens, with 11-year-olds to 13-year-olds less mature than older teens, and more likely "to endorse decisions that comply with what an authority seem to want as measured by their willingness to confess and plea bargain." Researchers suggest that these findings "point to the need for a broader legal construct of competency, one that recognizes that developmental factors – namely, cognitive and psychosocial immaturity – may compromise the critical decision-making ability of many young defendants in either adult or juvenile courts."[45] Other theorists identify additional questions concerning developmental competency based on data collected by the MacArthur Research Network. Katner[46] has suggested that these include whether newly identified diagnosable mental health issues of juveniles are accounted for in competency measures, how developmental immaturity, which often operates at a level comparable with disabled adults, should affect competency evaluations, and the effect of these 2 phenomena, diagnosable mental illness and developmental immaturity, on competency when combined.[46] Others have argued for revitalizing the infancy defense, which traditionally barred any liability for all children less than 7 years of age and for some children of limited maturity between the ages of 7 and 14 years.[47]

SUMMARY

The US Supreme Court's decisions in *Roper v Simmons* and *Graham v Florida*, invalidating the juvenile death penalty and sentences of LWOP for juveniles convicted of nonhomicide offenses, unavoidably invite further challenges to sentences of LWOP for juveniles convicted of homicides, and lengthy sentences for juveniles convicted of all offenses, because both types of punishment ignore the cognitive, psychosocial, and neuroanatomic distinctiveness of juveniles that the Court recognized in *Roper* and *Graham*.

REFERENCES

1. In re Gault, 387 US 1, 31–57 (1967).
2. In re Winship, 397 US 358 (1970).
3. Breed v. Jones, 421 US 519 (1975).
4. McKeiver v. Pennsylvania, 403 US 528 (1971).
5. Kent v. United States, 383 US 541 (1966).
6. Eddings v. Oklahoma, 455 US 104 (1982).
7. Thompson v. Oklahoma, 487 US 815 (1988).
8. Stanford v. Kentucky and Wilkins v. Missouri, 492 US 361 (1989).
9. Lewis DO, Pincus JH, Bard B, et al. Neuropsychiatric, psychoeducational, and family characteristics of 14 juveniles condemned to death in the United States. Am J Psychiatry 1988;145:584–9.
10. Roper v. Simmons, 543 US 551 (2005).
11. Graham v. Florida, 560 US ___, 130 S.Ct. 2011 (2010).
12. US Const., Amend. VIII.
13. Harmelin v. Michigan, 501 US 957 (1991).
14. Ewing v. California, 538 US 11 (2003).

15. Naovarath v. Nevada, 105 Nevada 525, 779 P2d 944 (1989).
16. Workman v. Commonwealth, 429 SW2d 374 (Ky 1968).
17. Harris v. Wright, 93 F3d 581 (9th Cir 1996).
18. State v. Pilcher, 655 So2d 636 (La.App 1995).
19. Tate v. Florida, 864 So2d 44 (Fla. App. 4th Dist 2003).
20. Trop v. Dulles, 356 US 86 (1958).
21. Weems v. United States, 217 US 349 (1910).
22. Robinson v. California, 370 US 660 (1962).
23. Enmund v. Florida, 458 US 782 (1982).
24. Coker v. Georgia, 433 US 584 (1977).
25. Kennedy v. Louisiana, 554 US 407, 128 S.Ct. 2641 (2010).
26. Atkins v. Virginia, 536 US 304 (2002).
27. Penry v. Lynaugh, 492 US 302 (1989).
28. State ex rel. Simmons v. Roper, 112 S.W.3d 397, 412 (Mo 2003).
29. 2004 WL 1636447, Brief for the American Psychological Association, and the Missouri Psychological Association as Amici Curiae Supporting Respondent (July 19, 2004).
30. 2004 WL 1633549 (US), Brief of the American Medical Association, American Psychiatric Association, American Society for Adolescent Psychiatry, American Academy of Child & Adolescent Psychiatry, American Academy of Psychiatry and the Law, National Association of Social Workers, Missouri Chapter of the National Association of Social Workers, and National Mental Health Association as Amici Curiae in Support of Respondent (July 16, 2004).
31. Arnett J. Reckless behavior in adolescence: a developmental perspective. Dev Rev 1992;12:339–73.
32. Steinberg L, Scott ES. Less guilty by reason of adolescence: developmental immaturity, diminished responsibility, and the juvenile death penalty. Am Psychol 2003;58:1009–14.
33. State of Florida v. Terrance Jamar Graham, 2007 WL 6600560 Circuit Court of Florida.
34. White HG, Frazier CE, Lanza-Kaduce L. A socio-legal history of Florida's juvenile transfer reforms. U Fla J L & Pub Pol'y 1999;10:249–75.
35. Scott ES. Criminal responsibility in adolescence: lessons from developmental psychology. In: Grisso T, Schwartz RG, editors. Youth on trial: a developmental perspective on juvenile justice. Chicago: University of Chicago; 2000. p. 291–324.
36. 2009 WL 2247127 (US), Brief for the American Medical Association and the American Academy of Child and Adolescent Psychiatry as Amici Curiae in Support of Neither Party (July 23, 2009).
37. 2009 WL 2236778 (US), Brief for the American Psychological Association, American Psychiatric Association, National Association of Social Workers, and Mental Health America As Amici Curiae Supporting Petitioners (July 23, 2009).
38. Miller v. State, ___ So.3d ___, 2010 WL 3377692, *8-*9 (Ala.Crim.App. 2010).
39. Jensen v. Zavaras, Slip Copy, 2010 WL 2825666 (D.Colo., July 16, 2010).
40. Greenholtz v. Inmates of Nebraska Penal and Correctional Complex, 442 US 1 (1979).
41. American Psychiatric Association. Adjudication of youths as adults in the criminal justice system. Position statement, approved by the Board of Trustees. 2005. Available at: http://www.psych.org/Departments/EDU/Library/APAOfficialDocumentsandRelated/PositionStatements/200507.aspx. Accessed April 11, 2011.

42. Grisso T. What do we know about youths' capacities as trial defendants. In: Grisso T, Schwartz RG, editors. Youth on trial: a developmental perspective on juvenile justice. Chicago: University of Chicago; 2000. p. 139–72.
43. Bonnie R. The competence of criminal defendants: a theoretical reformulation. Behav Sci Law 1992;10:291–316.
44. Available at: http://www.adjj.org. Accessed April 11, 2011.
45. MacArthur Foundation Research Network on Adolescent Development and Juvenile Justice. Adolescent legal competence in court. Available at: http://www.adjj.org/downloads/9805issue_brief_1.pdf. Accessed April 11, 2011.
46. Katner DR. The mental health paradigm and the Macarthur study: emerging issues challenging the competence of juveniles in delinquency systems. Am J Law Med 2006;32:503–83.
47. Kaban B, Orlando J. Revitalizing the infancy defense in the contemporary juvenile court. Rutgers Law Rev 2007;60:33–65.

Cornered: An Approach to School Bullying and Cyberbullying, and Forensic Implications

Jeff Q. Bostic, MD, EdD[a],*, Colby C. Brunt, JD[b]

KEYWORDS

• Bullying • Cyberbullying • Prevention • Forensic implications

The abuse of power, to intimidate and threaten others, will persist regardless of anti-bullying programs. Individuals of all ages aspire to define the rules by which we will all live, and will employ all available tactics within their repertoire, including intimidating others directly or indirectly, to push others to accede to their wishes. Schools work ardently to help individuals recognize the power of sharing and of considering the wishes of others, as this ultimately allows more individuals to attain what is good for them and for others. Schools similarly strive to cultivate repertoires of tactics for students to navigate diverse social interactions in mutually beneficial fashion. However, sometimes individuals will try to cut corners to accomplish their wants, often at the expense of others. Beyond simple manipulation, some individuals resort to intimidating or coercing others to obtain their wants.

BULLYING

In concrete terms, "bullying" is a legal conclusion whose definition varies between states. Recent Massachusetts legislation provides a comprehensive definition of bullying as

> *The repeated use by one or more students of a written, verbal or electronic expression or a physical act or gesture or any combination thereof, directed at a victim that: (i) causes physical or emotional harm to the victim or damage to the victim's property; (ii) places the victim in reasonable fear of harm to himself*

There was no financial support for this work.
The authors have nothing to disclose.
[a] Department of Psychiatry, Massachusetts General Hospital, Harvard Medical School, Boston, MA, USA
[b] Stoneman, Chandler and Miller, Boston, MA, USA
* Corresponding author.
E-mail address: jbostic@partners.org

Child Adolesc Psychiatric Clin N Am 20 (2011) 447–465
doi:10.1016/j.chc.2011.03.004
1056-4993/11/$ – see front matter © 2011 Elsevier Inc. All rights reserved.

childpsych.theclinics.com

or of damage to his property; (iii) creates a hostile environment at school for the victim; (iv) infringes on the rights of the victim at school; or (v) materially and substantially disrupts the education process or the orderly operation of a school.[1]

Bullying is often distinguished from "conflicts," whereby students of similar status (similar physical size, social status, and so forth) may have disputes and argue, but whereby one party does not have a decided unfair advantage over the other. Moreover, unlike typical conflicts, bullying tends to focus on the repeated actions by a student or students against a target.[2]

Bullying has become more visible in recent years, as several individual as well as school incidents have illuminated the pervasive damage that bullying has on students. Perhaps ironically, attention to bullying has increased markedly because bullied students themselves retaliated in prominent episodes of school violence in sites across the United States.[2–4] More recently, the P. Price case in Massachusetts has resulted in legislation designed to ensure that all Massachusetts schools recognize and address bullying behaviors across all domains of the students' lives. For example, the Massachusetts legislation has greatly expanded the ability of the school administration to respond to and address allegations of bullying that occur outside of school. Prior to this legislation, Massachusetts law provided limited means by which schools could intercede in bullying-like situations that occurred off campus or online. Under new law, school administrators can intervene on these matters and, if appropriate, take disciplinary action to address the bullying behavior. At present only two states, North Dakota and South Dakota, do not have legislation aimed at preventing bullying in schools, and approximately 32 of the 48 States with anti-bullying legislation have specific provisions addressing the use of cyberbullying (National Association of State Boards of Education).

Estimates over the past 5 years indicate that approximately one-third of students report being bullied over the past 6 months, compared with approximately one-seventh in 2001. Students who bully more often have externalizing disorders such as attention-deficit/hyperactivity disorder, while boys targeted for bullying more often have internalizing disorders such as anxiety or depression, or chronic somatic illnesses.[5] Targeted students report increased risks for developing depression, anxiety, suicidality, eating disorders, and somatic symptoms including headaches, stomachaches, colds, and sleep difficulties.[6] Targets also report decreased educational outcomes, including increased rates of truancy and disciplinary suspensions.[7]

Bullies also experience adverse risks. Although bullies seek status and may become "popular," bullies are no more "liked" than their "rejected" victims.[8] Over half of middle school bullies have criminal convictions by their early 20s.[9] Bullying has been associated with violent crimes, and with earlier onset of violent criminal offenses.[10] In addition, bullies are at increased risk for suicidal thoughts, attempts, and completions; one study found that targets had a 1.7-times increased risk of suicide attempts, whereas bullies had a 2.1-times increased risk (S. Hinduja, J.W. Patchin, www.cyberbullying.us).

Bystanders have been recognized as significant active participants in bullying situations, and no longer as simply passive observers.[11] Bystanders can reinforce the bully by laughing at the victim, assist the bully by joining in, or defend the victim, as well as act like an outsider, unaware or unconcerned by a bullying event.[12] Bystanders who observe bullying behaviors experience adverse effects as well. Bystanders describe greater distress by observing bullying than natural disasters or other life-threatening experiences.[13] However, bystanders who "defend" students are more likely to have personality traits of being agreeable and a prosocial orientation of trust, cooperation, and altruism.[14] Bystanders comprise not only students, but all the members of the system, such as teachers and staff.[15]

Perhaps most importantly, almost all students find themselves at various times in the role of a bully, victim, or bystander. While individuals may find themselves more frequently in one role than another, being in multiple roles is also associated with negative impacts such as increased suicidality.[16] Bullies and victims are both more likely than bystanders to describe feeling unsafe at school, and to feel sad most days. Bullies and bully-victims (playing both roles variously) feel "no good," and victims more often feel they "do not belong" at their school. The odds of becoming a victim decrease markedly as grade point average goes up.[17] These findings all illuminate that bullying is a relationship problem that requires relationship solutions.[18]

CYBERBULLYING

Cyberbullying is an emerging form of bullying by which students use electronic devices (eg, phone calls or text messages, emails, or postings on the Internet) to overpower others. Cyberbullying has become increasingly prominent over the past decade, and reveals subtle but significant changes in the nature of bullying, as more popular students have written or texted comments, often repetitively, ostracizing other students; historically, physically stronger students usually would stand off against smaller students. Cyberbullying affords several advantages over traditional bullying:

1. Comments or bullying messages can be constructed over time and not in the moment, giving the assailant the opportunity to orchestrate a more painful message and, should a targeted person respond, the bully can recruit others over time (and cyberspace) to construct further responses
2. Comments can often be "posted" or advanced anonymously or via pseudonyms
3. The assailant does not have to face the target, and can essentially "shoot from the bushes"
4. The assailant can titrate responses with much less fear of losing status among others; that is, in real-time situations, clever responses from the target, and interventions by bystanders or the system cannot be predicted in the moment; with cyberbullying the cyber-"space" between the participants minimizes immediate and clear intervention by relevant others
5. Cyberbullying relies on technology often unfamiliar to, and thus not monitored closely, by adults or school staff, and occurs largely outside their awareness, decreasing potential intervention by parents and staff
6. Cyberbullying allows individuals to configure their own rules of engagement to control the interaction with others and with minimal opportunities for detection and intervention by others, thus minimizing accountability or risks to the cyberbullies.

About half of all middle and high school students report being targets of cyberbullying, and one-third report cyberbullying others. Text messaging and cell-phone calling were the most frequent forms of cyberbullying. Cyberbullying episodes usually last approximately 1 week, and cyber victims appear to spend more time on the Internet than those less vulnerable to cyberbullying.[19] Cyber victims report feeling sad, angry, and depressed after being cyberbullied, indeed more so than the bullies.[20] Girls cyberbully more frequently because they do not have to be face to face with the target and can bully somewhat anonymously. Girls favor excluding other girls or making disparaging comments, whereas boys contend they are just "joking."[21] Most frequently, students will "name call" or "gossip" to bully others.[22] Efforts to get others to laugh at the target or to exclude the target are much more prominent than physical or direct verbal assaults. Girls report that they participate in "sexting" to attract others, yet most girls report they "sext" because of feeling coerced by male peers.[21] Boys are more likely to engage in verbal, physical, and cyberbullying, whereas girls are more likely to engage in social bullying and to be victims of cyberbullying.[23] Students who cyberbully are more likely to report moral disengagement and report lower justification or rationale for bullying their victims.[24]

Because students engage in cyberbullying largely outside of school, they do not perceive this as within the province of the school, or that school staff are helpful resources for addressing cyberbullying at school.[25] If cyberbullying is not addressed, it usually escalates and enters the school environment. Nevertheless, students will rarely report cyberbullying and, if they do, usually to a friend (approximately 30%) or a parent (<10%), but rarely to a school teacher or administrator (<5%).[21]

Case 1

A parent of a middle school student reported to the school administration that she saw a Facebook group that was created by other students entitled "I hate Jimmy Smith." The parent noticed this group when she was monitoring her own daughter's Facebook usage. Although her daughter was not a part of the group, the parent decided that she should contact the school to make them aware of the situation.

The student who was the subject of the group was also a middle school student who had Asperger's disorder. The administrators notified the student's parents of the web page. The school district also worked with the targeted student's parents to develop a safety plan to assist the student moving forward, and convened the special education team to look at any areas of the student's individual education plan that could be improved (eg, social pragmatic instruction).

The school then met with the creator of the Facebook page and his parents. The administration informed the student and his parents that this was brought to their attention by a community member, not the student who was the subject of the group or his parents. The administration stressed that this behavior was inappropriate and in violation of their student code of conduct regarding schooling. Although the actions of the student were beyond school grounds and not on the school's computers or server, the administration determined that because the behavior disrupted the targeted student at school, and with peers there, the administration imposed a multi-day suspension in accordance with the student handbook for disrespectful treatment of a peer.

The school administrators met with all the students who were members of the group and their parents to clarify the school's concern that students participated and contributed to a web page that declared their hatred of another classmate. These students were also disciplined in accordance with the code of conduct.

CONCEPTUAL APPROACH TO BULLYING

The current approach to bullying favors addressing 3 different participants in any bullying situation: the bully(ies), victims, and bystanders. As Olweus and Limber[4] have clarified, multiple roles (**Fig. 1**) further sophisticate this model. Specifically, "accomplices" may encourage or contribute to the bullying by laughing or by visually or verbally supporting the bully's comments or actions. Others may be active bystanders, ultimately reporting or acknowledging an incident, or they may be part

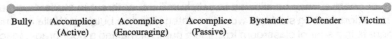

Fig. 1. The spectrum of bullying roles. (*Data from* Olweus D, Limber SP. Bullying in school: evaluation and dissemination of the Olweus Bullying Prevention Program. Am J Orthopsychiatry 2010;80(1):124–34.)

of the "target" group, but variously experience different levels of bullying. This triad model is illustrated in **Fig. 2**.

This model is helpful in distinguishing the individual roles in a social interaction; however, the social system in which an event occurs appears equally significant. In every situation, the social system within which the social interaction occurs provides some "set of rules," perhaps informal or malleable, that must be considered to clarify the context of possible bullying-type behaviors. William Golding's novel *Lord of the Flies* illuminates a quite primitive social situation whereby children, stranded on a remote island, form primitive teams that define the rules to govern social interactions and ultimately tease and even kill those who do not adhere, whereas schools adopt typically much more advanced and sophisticated systems. The empowered adults in schools (eg, principals, teachers) create, define, and model appropriate social interactions so that power differentials among students that favor intimidation or bullying are minimized. Nevertheless, in all social encounters children and adults stretch the roles of what is and is not acceptable, based on the "rules" of the system within which they are interacting, as they try to attain control within that setting. Accordingly, teachers and school staff can themselves be perceived as bullying students,[26] particularly those who suspend students more frequently or had been bullied themselves.[27] Teachers perceive physical and verbal aggression as more serious victimization than social exclusion, and teachers intervene when they feel sympathy for the victim and feel self-efficacy in dealing with bullying.[28,29] When confronted with bullying, teachers try to decide whether to punish the bullies, contact parents, foster coping skills in victims, or perform conflict resolution.[30] Even when targets enact commonly effective coping strategies, they often continue to be victimized.[31]

The significant problem, however, is that acceptable social behaviors, including the limits of what is intimidation or bullying, vary widely according to the specific setting. Settings within a school vary widely within the school day. Adults interpret and enforce the school's rules differently in the hall, the locker room, the cafeteria, and the playground. So "what works" in certain settings, such as classrooms, may not be the "rules" students enact in these other school settings across the day.[2] Moreover, the "rules" for student interactions may diverge from that modeled by the school staff;

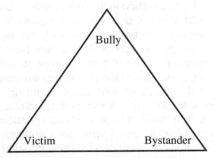

Fig. 2. Bullying roles: (1) Bully, (2) Victim, and (3) Bystander.

teachers or coaches may be allowed to yell, humiliate, or threaten students, whereas similar behaviors among students would be categorized as bullying. While it would be inappropriate in a school classroom to chide a pupil for making a poor grade, teachers sometimes perceive themselves as having different roles within the school system. School staff may be empowered in their school to model intimidation techniques, from singling out students in front of the class for poor performance to "yelling at" students on the sports field, including cultivating rituals to intimidate their opponents. This does not mean that all efforts to motivate students either in the classroom or on the athletic field should be "bully-proofed." The roles students and staff take during the day depends on the activity and the demands of the situation.

Case 2
A high school football team had what is commonly referred to as "hell week" during which student athletes participated in rigorous "2-a-day" workouts in preparation for potential season playoffs. The coaches used this time to build team camaraderie and work with the team on skills needed for high-pressure games. On the final night of "hell week" the senior boys made the freshman boys participate in various activities such as wearing dog collars, crawling on the field, and having things thrown at them while they crawled on the ground. Although the coaches were not present for this event, the coaches were aware of this "initiation" ritual and did nothing to condone or discourage this annual event.

The school administration became aware of this and interviewed the students who were involved. Although the freshman boys stated that it was just a part of "initiation" and that they were not complaining about what the upperclassmen did, the adminis-tration determined that the actions by the senior boys constituted "hazing." As such, the administration suspended the senior boys from games under the rules of the State interscholastic athletic association.

A senior's parents responded by filing for a court injunction to prevent the student's suspension for the upcoming game. The judge denied the injunction and let the prin-cipal's suspension stand, despite considerable outcry from the community, including parents of the freshman students who had been hazed. Many of the parents stated that the administration was overzealous in their actions toward the seniors, that this "behavior" was an accepted ritual on the football team, and finally that the students had resolved any conflict among them on their own and did not require the intervention of the school on this issue.

More importantly, what is acceptable at school, compared with "outside-school events" such as a sporting event, or within a neighborhood, vary widely in the "rules" that children are encouraged to practice in those social encounters. What is modeled and tolerated in one's neighborhood, or at a sporting event, may be in clear conflict with how the student is expected to behave at school; that is, the "rules" for school not only may not apply outside the school. The school rules may not "work," and indeed may leave students vulnerable if they attempt to employ what they have been asked to do at school, particularly if the school requires that students enact posi-tive comments toward each other such that students are not taught how to evade, resist, or change rules practiced in other social settings. Schoolchildren may well be confused about the limits of a "role" in diverse social situations for which they have not been prepared, and unable to enact what they are taught to do in a school when they are confronted with very different behaviors modeled by others, particularly adults who normally have the final say on the social rules in most settings.

The "system" defines the limits of behaviors in social interactions, and must be considered in all potential bullying situations (**Fig. 3**). For example, professional athletes, from boxers to football players, often attempt to intimidate one another, and this is rarely discouraged, particularly in professional sporting events. Moreover, during sporting events, most notably at the professional level, adults feel quite entitled to attempt to intimidate players (and other fans). In that social situation, the "rules" of bullying are drastically different than what would be tolerated in a kindergarten classroom or even playground. As long as the system supports or even tacitly encourages or just tolerates intimidation, at least in some social contexts, students will similarly replicate such bullying roles, as well as those of targets and bystanders, and the system may or may not intervene to restrict certain behaviors. So any model or approach to address bullying must recognize the system as another invested "participant," defining acceptable limits to exerting power over others, and sometimes intervening when those boundaries are transgressed. Much more importantly, students must be taught to recognize the various system "rules" they encounter, and how to extricate themselves from potentially distressing roles within these diverse systems.

System participation can be minimal, as it has not been acknowledged as a viable participant. In recent years, systems have been encouraged to participate in social interactions that allow power differentials to be exploited. Schools initially responded with "zero tolerance" policies, in which no evidence of bullying-type behavior would be "tolerated." Even the interpretation of this zero tolerance varies widely by systems, with some responding to any purported incident, and other systems contending that anyone "bullying" another will be disciplined or expelled. The irony of this latter interpretation of zero tolerance is that the system then "threatens" anyone who does not conform to the system's expectations and interpretations of the system's rules. One extreme example of this is that under the new State legislation, anyone can seek a restraining order against another individual for repeated bullying-like or harassing behavior. This change in the law will likely lead to an increase of student against student restraining orders; at present there is at least one instance where a teacher sought a restraining order against a student and ultimately the student was excluded from school for over 2 months as a result. While this may sometimes (rarely) be necessary, it remains a primitive response, counter to the opportunity inherent in schools, where skill development and practice can occur. Indeed, punishment tactics against bullying are ineffective and usually have the opposite result. School system responses that are effective for diminishing bullying clarify acceptable behaviors, making students accountable, while providing a supportive, caring environment rather than a punitive response. Punishing aggressors is less effective than providing new skills, promoting relationship building, and increasing awareness of bullying behaviors.[32]

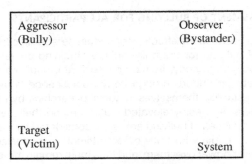

Fig. 3. Bullying roles: aggressor, target, observer, system.

Perhaps more importantly, rarely do individuals play only one role. In one school situation, a student may feel "targeted," whereas the same student in another classroom, recess, or lunchroom setting may feel powerful or only a perpetual bystander. The vitally important mission of a school is to provide tactics for students (and staff) when "cornered" into any role, so that these students can escape from cornered positions and navigate diverse social situations whereby they may feel bullied, paralyzed as a bystander, inclined to intimidate another, or empowered to enact a system response to a particular situation.

Case 3

A female fifth-grade charter school student, Jane, reported to her parents that her former friend, Annie, was making fun of her and hitting her in class when her teacher was not watching. Jane reported that Annie said that she was "only joking," but that Jane wanted Annie to stop. As a result, the parents contacted the school principal and requested that Annie be expelled.

The principal met with Annie to discuss the allegations from Jane. Annie denied that she did anything to Jane, and told the principal that it was Jane who was saying "mean things" to Annie while the teacher was not looking. Because the principal could not establish who was "bullying" whom, she met with both girls separately and together to discuss how to move forward and to encourage both of them to avoid contact with one another.

Shortly after meeting with the two girls, Jane's parents informed the principal that Annie continued to seek out Jane at school and would not leave her alone. In a small school with approximately 90 students, it was extremely difficult to ensure that the students would not run into each other in the halls, class, and so forth. Forced with a difficult situation, the principal met again with the students to discuss their not contacting one another. Jane's parents threatened the school that they would seek a restraining order against Annie if this behavior continued, requested that Annie be expelled, and that they be informed of all actions that the school might take regarding its discipline of Annie. The principal informed the parents that they could not release any information regarding another student to them, and that they could only inform the parents that they were acting in accordance with the school's code of conduct. Ultimately, Jane's parents did not seek a restraining order, but rather requested that Jane be moved to another classroom.

The situation between the two students dissipated with time and, perhaps, as a result of the switch in classroom placement. However, because of the threatened legal action by Jane's parents, the school had legal counsel conduct a district-wide training for staff to alert them to relevant anti-bullying legislation and to institute a bullying policy curriculum for all students.

FUNCTIONAL ASSESSMENT OF BULLYING FOR ALL PARTICIPANTS

Bullying is employed because it is effective for certain persons in certain situations. The potential benefits of bullying for the bully include obtaining power over other peers, obtaining desired objects (money, items, and so forth), and deference from others (**Table 1**). During late childhood through early adolescence, when bullying peaks, students who bully establish themselves in social hierarchies by demonstrating their dominance over peers, and enjoy elevated status among their peers.[33,34] However, the long-term consequences of bullying are rarely considered by students who initiate bullying interactions. People who bully others ultimately recognize that others may amass and exert similar power over them, and thus must remain more attentive, in every social encounter, both of the rules of that social situation (school, work, and so forth),

Table 1
Functional assessment of bullying for all participants

Role	Potential Benefits of Bullying (What Sustains Bullying)	Long-Term Impacts of Bullying On:
Aggressor (bully)	Control over others; setting the "rules" to advantage themselves over others	Retaliation by others; conduct disorder; fear of "dethronement" by others
Target (victim)	Learn to toughen up; recognize what makes them a target and motivation for change	Fear, distrust of others and the system, increased anxiety, depression; retreat from social situations; posttraumatic stress disorder (PTSD)
Observer (bystander)	Recognize socially desirable and targeted behaviors; passive to active enjoyment of watching weaker individuals sanctioned by aggressors or the system; ability to accept, tolerate, or avoid distressing situations	Dexterity at avoiding involvement; desensitized to others being abused; powerlessness, anxiety, depression, PTSD (about observed traumatic encounters); guilt about actions not taken
System	Preservation of social order and hierarchy; tacit enforcement of social roles and differentiated power between students; tacit sanctioning of troublesome students; preservation of system resources as aggressors establish order	Galvanizing of a school culture difficult to alter; definition of how students are viewed, protected, and taught within a school culture; prideful identity within the larger school and local community

and of the potential adversaries "stronger" than them. Aggressive behavior crossing into bullying is reinforced by others, within and outside schools, who encourage such students to intimidate others in the classroom or through school activities or sports.

Ultimately, social interactions collapse when individuals finds themselves relegated to any corner of this triangle or square. The aggressors may be most committed to preserving these roles, and perceive the most benefit, but as the saying goes, "if it ain't good for both, it ain't good for long." So in the vast majority of cases someone seeks an alternative course; the aggressors may seek to widen their influence to additional students. The targets may avoid being in environments where the aggressor is likely to appear, or deny that they are actually being bullied and instead contend it is a joking relationship. Observers may ultimately access others or, more rarely, intervene. The system is ultimately the party best positioned to effect meaningful changes in these roles, but usually does not seek out events or intervene unless a problem is identified to the system.

Aggressors

Students trapped in these corners experience largely negative outcomes in both the immediate circumstance and long-term impact. Aggressors may briefly feel empowered, or obtain items from their targets, but may become more aware of ultimate consequences including system intervention. Accordingly, aggressors either experience reinforcement for their behaviors and continue and exaggerate these behaviors, which are largely antisocial, toward crystallization of conduct disorder symptoms, or experience increased fear of ultimate retaliation by the system. Fundamentally for aggressors, social encounters are based on who can overpower the other. Mutual beneficial relationships and tactics for working together are not reinforced, and thus less likely are internalized for aggressors. Aggressors are left with a primitive, negative approach to social encounters and all others. Aggressors are more vulnerable to conduct disorder and incarceration than others, as well as dysfunctional relationships with peers.

Targets

Targets are vulnerable to feeling powerless, and perhaps more importantly, to seeing themselves as targets for some reason; that is, targets may attempt to construe bullying events into "playful teasing," but this rarely sustains, and ultimately others similarly clarify the true nature of these roles. Moreover, the target is vulnerable to experiencing this role in other social encounters and may not perceive being weak, but act differently in new social encounters based on past experience. Targets are more likely than other students to feel anxious and depressed, and are inclined to develop clinical symptoms of anxiety and depressive disorders, in many instances culminating in developing "school phobia." Complicating this, however, is that targets may sometimes also have psychiatric disorders, from pervasive developmental disorders to internalizing or externalizing disorders, which may allow them to appear weaker, or to "stick out" such that the aggressor feels socially encouraged to address atypical behaviors.

Observers

Observers are similarly positioned for negative outcomes. Observers usually feel distressed by watching injustices, and fear being both targeted themselves and paralyzed to respond so that the bullying stops. Approximately 80% of bullying events occur in front of peers, yet fewer than 20% of bystanders intervene.[35] Accordingly, observers tend to avoid participation, or may employ tactics to diminish the intensity of discomfort by making bullying encounters into playful episodes, justifying the aggressor's acknowledgment of the target's behaviors that warrant comment by others, or minimizing the impact of the episode on the participants. Moreover, observers may fail to alter subsequent encounters, and feel increasingly guilty as well as anchored in their role as passive observer without the means or skills to alter this event or any events in other circumstances. Observers may experience anxiety and depression, and galvanize defenses that favor denial over intervention.

The System

The system itself may be traumatized by bullying episodes. Those expected to provide safe circumstances and are empowered to provide skills to enhance students' lives may feel disconnected, disavowed, and impotent in creating a positive culture in their schools. Systems may overreact in angry or punitive fashion, leading aggressors to be more selective about where and how they enact bullying, but without making significant changes in the school's culture. Systems may similarly avoid or minimize episodes, because addressing bullying requires significant time and intervention with aggressors, targets, observers, and parents, usually apart from the school's already overwhelmed staff, resources, and educational expectations.

Case 4

A group of high school students "staged" a fight in the school cafeteria. No one was harmed, and the teachers who were present saw no need to take action to stop the "fight" or report any of the students involved to administration. Shortly after the incident, a student who taped the incident on her cell phone uploaded it to a social networking site. In the background of the video, the student taping the incident could be heard narrating the event. At one point, the student was heard to use terms such as "snitches" and "bitches."

Within a few hours of the video being posted online, the administration was made aware of the video, and suspended the student who filmed the incident and used "offensive language." The administration then interviewed all the students involved to clarify who was involved in the planning of the event, and what they each knew about the event. Ultimately the administration disciplined more than 20 students for their involvement of the staged fight and for the dissemination of the staged fight on the Internet, due to it being determined that these actions substantially disturbed the school environment.

Shortly after the incident was reported in the local media, community members, including members of the school board, called for the expulsion of the student who had taped and uploaded the staged fight to the social networking site. Ultimately, the administration resisted social pressures to take any further disciplinary action against the student who uploaded the video or any other student involved. No one raised concerns about the teachers who witnessed the event and did not intervene. The administrators recognized that too much ambiguity existed in their school policies regarding students using their cell phones at school, even outside of classes, and a lack of clarity about student privacy rights that precluded disseminating photos or videos over the Internet or texting without student and parent consent. In addition, the school recognized a need for contextualizing student behaviors, as the offensive language appeared to be recitation of a popular song lyric among students. School staff reviewed opportunities and specific recommendations to help students recognize appropriate behaviors at school, regardless of what students might see modeled on popular television shows, even PG-rated movies, and on radio airwaves.

EFFECTIVE BULLYING PREVENTION PROGRAMS

The foremost principle in developing an effective anti-bullying program for any school is to define, practice, and reinforce the "rules of social encounters" within the school system, and to advocate how and why these rules are preferable for social relationships in other situations (**Table 2**). If the school rules are not internally embraced, students will perceive that these rules are hollow and unhelpful in the wider world. Just as unfortunate, if the rules do not yield more beneficial social encounters among diverse individuals, they will not be valued or attempted in other situations, and instead be quickly forgotten. Accordingly, the policies that surround the desired interactions between students, between staff, between students and staff, and between staff and parents should be carefully examined, and appropriate policies devised and implemented. The implementation requires that the school system identify desirable behaviors through specific policies, and more importantly, model desirable behavior. Several programs conducive to prosocial interactions and to anti-bullying exist, such as Positive Behavioral Intervention Support (PBIS) and the Olweus anti-bullying program.[4] While extrapolating these programs has sometimes had mixed results,[36] almost all effective programs focus on the interactions of everyone within the school.

Olweus and Limber[4] have, over the course of approximately 25 years, identified program components important in reducing bullying, and categorized them at the level of the school, classroom, individual, and community. At the school level, having staff discussions about bullying, including parents, and introducing bullying rules appear important. At the classroom level, posting and enforcing anti-bullying rules, and having frequent meetings with students and families have been important. At the individual

Table 2
Developmentally sensitive techniques to move out of the corners

	Technique	Elementary School	Middle School	High School
System (school)	Clarify rules for system	Determine the guiding principles for social interaction, importance of democratic participation vs structured control	Specify how "diverse" or unusual students will be treated, or if students do unusual acts; clarify the inclusion vs exclusion "rules" of the school and how they actually operate	Clarify how the rules apply to specific situations; provide hypothetical scenarios and encourage students to comment on options, consequences
	Create policy	Create and circulate policy to invest staff, students, and parents in the "rules"	Query staff, and identify priorities to optimize the school culture and to minimize ostracism	Rely on staff and students to identify helpful policy and procedures, and ensure they are well known in the building
	Respond to allegations	Determine the process for responding to bullying incidents, and remain consistent in following up and/or fine-tuning the policy	Determine the process for responding to bullying incidents and monitor outcomes for all parties	Clarify the process for responding to bullying events and apply it judiciously, being mindful of what principles you are seeking to teach
	Create feedback loop	Identify mechanisms for staff, students, and parents to continuously comment on potential bulling events, as well as school "rules"	Identify mechanisms for staff, students, and parents to continuously comment on potential bulling events, as well as school "rules"	Ensure that students and staff are regularly involved in evaluating the bullying events, and the policies designed to improve school interactions
Aggressor (bully)	Ally rather than intimidate	What makes good friends? How to find what others are good at that may enrich your life	Recognize that group configurations change each week, and benefits/risks of including various individuals	Recognize that others can be helpful contributors to one's missions and interests
	Use power for good	How to make others feel good, and enjoying their moments	Include others who may feel disenfranchised; model how to lead	Examination of larger circles of influence and impacts on the world
	Treat as want to be treated	Consider how others feel and how	Examine impacts on those excluded; identify what is wanted by being in control and empowerment by others	Examine how everyone should be treated for most people to feel positively
	Identify what's triggering	Examine antecedents to aggressive behaviors and alternatives to feel comfortable	Clarify what provokes aggressive behaviors, and the impacts then, and later, on others	Examine deeper desires of the aggressor, and what long-term impacts on both self and others are most probable

Target (victim)			
Confront aggressor	How to tell aggressors to stop current comments	Tell aggressors how to speak differently to them	Label inappropriate comments by the aggressor
Change topic	Shift the conversation if it is uncomfortable	Redirect the conversation to appropriate topics or away from condescension	Offer conversations you will participate in, or relevant appropriate topics
Ignore aggressor	Look away, talk to others, walk away	Avoid gossip or actions that escalate conflict, and instead minimize support for aggressors	Engage or comment about useful topics; clarify that you will leave the situation if the aggressor persists
Access peers	Look at friends to see their reactions; ask friends to play with you	Identify different groupings of peers, which ones are of like mind to you, and other groups/members who may have helpful input	Ask peers for their perceptions and suggestions; look to peer allies for support to visit or engage the aggressor
Access adults	Identify helpful adults, how to tell vs "tattle"	Identify adults aware of the group "rules" in the school; seek input and appropriate actions vs just "telling on/snitching"	Seek input from adults, using hypothetical situations and courses of action if feasible, or identifying the range of students affected by bullying
Observer (bystander)			
Check reactions of others	Look to see others' reactions	Examine the reactions of different students and student groups	Examine and seek perceptions of others to navigate bullying situations
Intervene by taking positive steps	Step in, alone or with others, to confront the aggressor or to include the target	Step in, alone or with others, to address the aggressor, mindful of various group rules or dynamics	Invoke humor, redirection to the good intentions gone awry, and win-win opportunities for all parties
Change interaction	Change the topic or "game" to something more comfortable	Shift the conversation, disallow singling out a student, refocus on the larger school rules or objectives	Shift the conversation or activity, label what you are observing, suggest alternatives to have an appropriate, more productive talk
Access adults	Identify helpful adults; describe facts accurately to adults, and seek input and action	Identify helpful, aware adults; seek input on options to alter the situation, including adult intervention	Identify useful adults, seek their perceptions and suggestion; discuss your options with them

level, supervision of student activities, meeting with students, parents, and staff, and developing plans for affected students appear helpful. Community interventions to cultivate community partnerships and to spread anti-bullying throughout the community appear effective.

Several school variables are associated with decreases in bullying. These variables include effective school leadership, professional development involving all parents and school personnel (including cafeteria staff, bus drivers, secretaries, and so forth), access to mental health services for aggressors and targets, classroom curricula to educate students to recognize bullying, bystander tactics to support victims, anger management, assertiveness training, conflict resolution, and perspective-taking. Similarly, effective school policies increase adult supervision and foster school norms against bullying by promoting "consistent, fair, and nonpunitive consequences for violations." Pepler has advocated a developmental-system view toward bullying, focusing on the social architecture sustaining the bullying, and also the scaffolding of interventions with the individuals involved in particular incidents.[37]

TACTICS TO GET OUT OF THE CORNERS

Techniques to help students (and staff) move out of corners is essential teaching for everyone in the system. These techniques afford students specific strategies and skills necessary to not only move away from undesirable roles in their specific school situations, but more importantly to draw on the "rules" of a system when in other situations or circumstances where they find themselves "cornered" outside of school into the role of bully, victim, or bystander. These techniques vary according to the developmental status of the students as well as the developmental status of the system itself. Younger, more primitive students and systems require different tactics than older students or more advanced systems. These techniques are provided in **Table 2**.

Elementary School

The primary principle at this level is to teach children the appropriate rules for social interactions as though these students have not been exposed to such discussions previously. While most children have been taught sharing, being respectful to others, and so forth, these children may not have been in larger social systems such as a school where the child's own home rules may not be quite the same. Students may be familiar with "home rules," or lack of them, or how to manipulate them, and resist replacing these rules with more restrictive or higher-expectation school rules. Efforts to teach children the rules of engagement, as though the child is *tabula rasa* (a "blank slate"), is appropriate at this phase of their development.

In concrete terms, staff cohesion on the rules and priorities requires ongoing attention and review. At this level, students are neither familiar with rules nor socially encouraged to identify incongruities, leaving these students with little impact on what teachers implement. Accordingly, close teacher observation by other teachers and administrators is important to determine whether teachers are actually implementing what is desired. In addition, students need clear review of the rules (and presence of the rules, stated positively, in multiple places throughout the school). Most importantly, connections between the rules and real-life events help students to extrapolate rules to real-life situations, and to rely on these rules for guiding their decision making. Teachers' descriptions of real-life examples may help students to "see" the rationale and impacts of these rules in given situations. In addition, the community, or parent "buy-in" is a key component at this stage to encourage the carry-over of these "life lessons" between the home and the school. As such, including the parents as stakeholders in any anti-bullying curriculum will help obtain overall success by fostering the values espoused by an anti-bullying curriculum with the families.

Middle School

The fundamental principle at the middle school level is that students elevate loyalty to each other over the rules identified by adults. That is, students more fear "snitching" or betraying each other than they do defying or breaking a school rule. Efforts mindful of this developmental shift are necessary to counter adolescents' efforts to prove their independence from adults and to create their own social rules.

In concrete terms, adolescents can be taught to examine the reactions of peers to potential bullying efforts. For males, these events are often considered "joking" or "playing around," and may not be recognized as intimidating or distressful to others. Teaching all adolescents to identify when something is hurtful, whether intended as funny or not, is a skill they will all need for the remainder of their lives. Being able to not laugh along with others, to counter that what is said to them does not feel funny to them, and even walking away are vital skills when in this situation. In addition, others proximate to these bullying encounters may exaggerate an observer role by looking away or denying the event at that time, as they feel powerless to respond or intervene. Accordingly, practicing responding to events by labeling them, and using the good intention gone awry, may allow observing adolescents to intervene with less risk of becoming targets themselves. Stating "It looks like you guys are trying to be funny, but it's not coming off that way," identifies and creates a conflict in the mind of the aggressor(s), who may think their behavior garners them esteem among peers.

Most importantly, teaching adolescents how to access adults is the most vital, yet difficult, skill needed to reduce bullying behaviors at this level. Certain techniques, such as allying a friend or responding to the aggressor, seem to be more effective than crying or appearing weak, although the research has remained inconsistent. Any reaching out to an adult is verification that the student is not "independent," so students actively resist engaging adults. Accordingly, schools have to make explicit, by policies and by actions, that accessing others is a useful, appropriate technique when confronted with a difficult situation. To do this, initial policy descriptions that address the difficulty adolescents have in accessing adults can help, and rationales may be helpful to "complicate the adolescents' thinking," so that the adolescent is more receptive to doing something unfamiliar (and better than the usual "handle it my own, or by accessing my peers"). Rationales include "if you had gone swimming in a place where you had been told not to go by adults, and your friend started to drown, would you access adults?" Most adolescents can recognize that life-or-death events require admitting they do not have a necessary skill, so they similarly can be taught to recognize that many unusual circumstances will arise during adolescence that will be distressing to them. The essential tactic of accessing other peers, or adults if events are not going well, can be adapted by encouraging adolescents to approach preferred adults (eg, teachers, parents, staff, and so forth) even to describe "hypothetical events" (ie, the circumstances that they are in, or observing, or enacting, but that make them feel uncomfortable) to others to identify different options for addressing issues. Helping adolescents to recognize that effective adults seek input and support and that this is not a sign of dependence on adults or a weakness is among the most important strategies to cultivate a school climate in which bullying becomes visible and is addressed. Similarly, adults must also "walk this walk," by seeking input from adolescents on diverse topics to model that accessing others is not a show of inadequacy or weakness.

High School (and College)

The primary principle in higher grades is to help students recognize that consideration and inclusion of others is much more effective for social stability than intimidation and exclusion. All students contribute to the social system they are a part of, and can contribute to ongoing "caste" efforts by others, or to "inclusion" of others, which requires patience and tolerance of that which may be unfamiliar. So every action (or inaction) of these students affects the rules that define that social system. If students allow other students to intimidate or bully others, then in-groups and out-groups will hierarchically organize, leaving a few students in the upper "caste," but the majority in subservient, "less valued" roles, usually having nothing to do with the students' actual ability to contribute to the school.

In concrete terms, clarifying higher principles that lead to successful coexistence, in contrast to ongoing tribal fears of another group infringing or competing, is necessary to help students think beyond their own immediate needs. Student desires for autonomy, a carry-over developmental task from adolescence, may conflict with impositions of any type from adults. Efforts to expand adolescents' recognition of not only alternatives available in given situations but also probable consequences affecting them, and others, for choosing a particular option may improve wider, more prosocial, and altruistic actions by these students. Sensitivity to what is acceptable in given environments, and to what impedes potential, unnecessary conflicts becomes an increasingly necessary skill for adolescents to navigate independently diverse circumstances.

Cyberbullying

The aforementioned tactics similarly apply to cyberbullying. However, the nature of cyberbullying necessitates some additional interventions. Parental support decreases bullying victimization, although parents usually perceive that they are far more aware and restrictive of their child's media diet than they actually are.[23]

Parental and school awareness of child/student media use, and inquiry about, as well as monitoring of, media use remains important. Again, developmental differences remain important, as privacy becomes increasingly important as children reach middle school, and resist parental knowledge of media use. Nevertheless, ongoing inquiries by parents, perhaps performed in displacement, may allow these topics to be more easily discussed with an adolescent. (For example, "I read/saw/heard about a child who had been receiving hostile text messages. What would you say to that student?" Or, "What would you wish that someone would do if you were in that situation?") Schools can similarly equip staff with familiarity about cyberbullying and tactics to provide to students and families. Indeed, schools can be helpful in teaching students appropriate use of media, including texting from cell phones or students' participation in video games, rather than react when students "guess" what might or might not be appropriate uses of various media. Thus, school policy efforts to clarify appropriate use of media as it affects school participation (including cyberbullying) is an effective proactive "system" function to enhance appropriate student cyber behavior.

In addition, cyberbullying is by its nature a different form of bullying, requiring different responses to students in roles already described. The most effective responses for those being cyberbullied is to simply "de-friend" someone on a social network site, or to abort the conversation. The transition from "getting the last word" (continuing the e-chat) to "walking away" (stopping the e-conversation and avoiding the e-bully) becomes an important, and valuable, strategy for students to learn to employ and access amidst these types of episodes, particularly as cyber aggressors may be unknown and much older than physically present cyberbullies. That is, the longer the texting continues, the greater the probability of escalation as compared with the face-to-face encounter, but perhaps worse, the greater the probability of "widening the circle" to create essentially "cybergangbullying" between students, not only increasing the conflicts among others but lengthening the episode. Similarly, assisting students pursuing cyberbullying-type behaviors may benefit from being provided alternative tactics to address and resolve conflicts with other students rather than assail students from the "cyberweeds." In addition, education for observers to identify and address inappropriate cyber comments, and without escalating conflicts as already described, often requires tactics beyond what usually works in face-to-face encounters. Specifically, observer labeling of inappropriate cyber language or conversations, efforts supportive of appropriate interactions face to face or via media, and modeling appropriate cyber behaviors may be most helpful. It is clear that differences in nuance, both developmentally and unique to emerging media, will continue to require additional policies and specific tactics to keep up with the unanticipated opportunities for social interactions, positive and negative, available through diverse media.

SUMMARY

Bullying is often more subtle than is portrayed. Students often shift among and between roles, depending on the circumstances and who else is present. Even more confusing, the socially acceptable behaviors in various environments have become even more difficult for children to employ as more behaviors are modeled through students' ever-expanding media diets, which include more extreme depictions, normalizing such behaviors for students. Video games have indeed been developed that specifically allow participants to take the role of "bully" and to terrorize others.[2]

The system should be included as an equal player in bullying scenarios, with an obligation to clarify the rules of social encounters in that setting, to ensure that all participants (students, teachers, staff) in that system practice those rules, and to address inappropriate violations by assisting all affected participants with useful, feasible alternatives when in a distressing situation.

Developmental considerations must be included in devising means for students and staff to identify and address bullying behaviors. Students will require developmentally sensitive strategies to respond to bullying incidents, both within and beyond the confines of the school itself. Because many, if not most, bullying events reveal multiple and subtle difficulties affecting multiple students, school efforts to help students recognize bullying behaviors and to practice strategies to evade distressing roles is well suited to the purview of the school.

REFERENCES

1. Massachusetts General Laws, Chapter 71 Section 37 O(a).
2. Barboza GE, Schiamberg LB, Oehmke J, et al. Individual characteristics and the multiple contexts of adolescent bullying: an ecological perspective. J Youth Adolesc 2009;38(1):101–21.
3. Williams K, Rivera L, Neighbours R, et al. Youth violence prevention comes of age: research, training and future directions. Annu Rev Public Health 2007;28: 195–211.
4. Olweus D, Limber SP. Bullying in school: evaluation and dissemination of the Olweus Bullying Prevention Program. Am J Orthopsychiatry 2010;80(1):124–34.
5. Luukkonen AH, Rasanen P, Hakko H, et al. Bullying behavior in relation to psychiatric disorders and physical health among adolescents: a clinical cohort of 508

underage inpatient adolescents in Northern Finland. Psychiatry Res 2010;178(1): 166–70.

6. Fekkes M, Pijpers FI, Verloove-Vanhorick SP. Bullying behavior and associations with psychosomatic complaints and depression in victims. J Pediatr 2004;144(1): 17–22.

7. DeVoe JF, Kaffenberger S. Student reports of bullying: results from the 2001 school crime supplement to the national crime victimization survey (NCES 2005–310). U.S. Department of Education, National Center for Education Statistics. Washington, DC: U.S. Government Printing Office; 2005. p. 1–30.

8. Sijtsema JJ, Veenstra R, Lindenberg S, et al. Empirical test of bullies' status goals: assessing direct goals, aggression, and prestige. Aggress Behav 2009;35(1):57–67.

9. Macklem G. Bullying and teasing: social power in children's groups. New York: Plenum; 2003.

10. Luukkonen AH, Riala K, Hakko H, et al. Bullying behaviour and criminality: a population-based follow-up study of adolescent psychiatric inpatients in Northern Finland. Forensic Sci Int 2011;207(1–3):106–10.

11. Twemlow SW, Fonagy P, Sacco FC. The role of the bystander in the social architecture of bullying and violence in schools and communities. Ann N Y Acad Sci 2004;1036:215–32.

12. Salmivalli C. Participant role approach to school bullying: implications for interventions. J Adolesc 1999;22(4):453–9.

13. Janson GR, Hazler RJ. Trauma reactions of bystanders and victims to repetitive abuse experiences. Violence Vict 2004;19(2):239–55.

14. Tani F, Greenman PS, Schneider BH, et al. Bullying and the big five. Sch Psychol Int 2003;24:131–46.

15. Stueve A, Dash K, O'Donnell L, et al. Rethinking the bystander role in school violence prevention. Health Promot Pract 2006;7(1):117–24.

16. Rivers I, Noret N. Participant roles in bullying behavior and their association with thoughts of ending one's life. Crisis 2010;31(3):143–8.

17. Glew GM, Fan MY, Katon W, et al. Bullying and school safety. J Pediatr 2008; 152(1):123–8, 128 e121.

18. Pepler D, Jiang D, Craig W, et al. Developmental trajectories of bullying and associated factors. Child Dev 2008;79(2):325–38.

19. Smith PK, Mahdavi J, Carvalho M, et al. Cyberbullying: its nature and impact in secondary school pupils. J Child Psychol Psychiatry 2008;49(4):376–85.

20. Mishna F, Cook C, Gadalla T, et al. Cyber bullying behaviors among middle and high school students. Am J Orthopsychiatry 2010;80(3):362–74.

21. Snell PA, Englander EK. Cyberbullying victimization and behaviors among girls: applying research findings in the field. J Soc Sci 2010;6:510–4.

22. Dehue F, Bolman C, Vollink T. Cyberbullying: youngsters' experiences and parental perception. Cyberpsychol Behav 2008;11(2):217–23.

23. Wang J, Iannotti RJ, Nansel TR. School bullying among adolescents in the United States: physical, verbal, relational, and cyber. J Adolesc Health 2009;45(4): 368–75.

24. Pornari CD, Wood J. Peer and cyber aggression in secondary school students: the role of moral disengagement, hostile attribution bias, and outcome expectancies. Aggress Behav 2010;36(2):81–94.

25. Agatston PW, Kowalski R, Limber S. Students' perspectives on cyber bullying. J Adolesc Health 2007;41(6 Suppl 1):S59–60.

26. Twemlow SW, Fonagy P, Sacco FC, et al. Teachers who bully students: a hidden trauma. Int J Soc Psychiatry 2006;52(3):187–98.

27. Twemlow SW, Fonagy P. The prevalence of teachers who bully students in schools with differing levels of behavioral problems. Am J Psychiatry 2005; 162(12):2387–9.
28. Yoon J, Kerber K. Bullying: elementary teachers' attitudes and intervention strategies. Res Educ 2003;69:27–35.
29. Yoon J. Predicting teacher interventions in bullying situations. Educ Treat Children 2004;27(1):37–45.
30. Limber S, Espelage D, Swearer S, editors. Bullying in American schools: a social-ecological perspective on prevention and intervention. Mahwah (NJ): Erlbaum; 2004.
31. Kochenderfer-Ladd B, Skinner K. Children's coping strategies: moderators of the effects of peer victimization? Dev Psychol 2002;38(2):267–78.
32. Olweus D. Bullying at school: basic facts and effects of a school based intervention program. J Child Psychol Psychiatry 1994;35(7):1171–90.
33. Pellegrini A, Bartini M. A longitudinal study of bullying, victimization, and peer affiliation during the transition from primary school to middle school. Am Educ Res J 2000;39:699–725.
34. Rodkin PC, Hodges EV. Bullies and victims in the peer ecology: four questions for psychologists and school professionals. Sch Psychol Rev 2003;32:384–400.
35. Nickerson AB, Mele D, Princiotta D. Attachment and empathy as predictors of roles as defenders or outsiders in bullying interactions. J Sch Psychol 2008; 46(6):687–703.
36. Bauer NS, Lozano P, Rivara FP. The effectiveness of the Olweus Bullying Prevention Program in public middle schools: a controlled trial. J Adolesc Health 2007; 40(3):266–74.
37. Pepler DJ. Bullying interventions: a binocular perspective. J Can Acad Child Adolesc Psychiatry 2006;15(1):16–20.

Children of Divorce: The Differential Diagnosis of Contact Refusal

Bradley W. Freeman, MD

KEYWORDS

- Divorce • Contact refusal • Alienation • Child custody
- Children and adolescents

Marriages in the United States are certainly not a stranger to divorce and all the related psychosocial issues involved. The Centers for Disease Control and Prevention estimates that the divorce rate over the past few years has been essentially half the rate of marriages.[1] Children involved in divorce have a wide range of experiences and outcomes related to the nature of the divorce, their own resilience and coping skills, and the available support network both during the separation and after. Research has demonstrated that children of divorced parents tend to exhibit more psychopathology than children of intact families.[2] This finding does not imply that all divorces are harmful to children, but divorce is a significant stressor, for good or bad, on the psychological health of the children involved.

The relationship between the divorcing parents can also range from amicable to one of great hostility and vindictiveness. This postdivorce relationship continues to have a profound effect on the mental health of the children.[3] Depending on the developmental stage of the child, divorce can be experienced in several ways. Children respond to this change differently. One particular area that the children are forced to restructure is their relationship with the parents, especially a noncustodial parent. Some children tolerate this change well, whereas others exhibit maladaptive behaviors, including contact refusal. This article discusses some of the reasons for a child to refuse contact with a parent after divorce and potential therapeutic interventions, which have important implications in several areas, the most obvious being custody disputes.

CONTACT REFUSAL

In the most general sense, contact refusal is a behavior in which a child resists spending time with a parent. Because there are many different causes for this

Dr Freeman has nothing to disclose.
Department of Psychiatry, Vanderbilt University School of Medicine, 1601 23rd Avenue South, Suite 3050, Nashville, TN 37212, USA
E-mail address: bradley.w.freeman@vanderbilt.edu

Child Adolesc Psychiatric Clin N Am 20 (2011) 467–477
doi:10.1016/j.chc.2011.03.008
1056-4993/11/$ – see front matter © 2011 Elsevier Inc. All rights reserved.

behavior, it should not be assumed that the child dislikes the parent or that the parent is unfit. The term contact refers to physical approximation and various methods of communication. Some children become resistant to even discussing the parent with a third party or having pictures of the parent in their environment. The term refusal corresponds to a willful choice, a decision, made by the child. In other words, a situation in which a parent does not allow a child to visit the noncustodial parent is not a form of contact refusal. The child must be the one who is resistant.

In addition to the determination of a child's custody and visitation arrangements, contact refusal by a child toward a particular parent or caregiver might relate to parental rights, the child's own autonomy, and the enforcement of court-mandated visitation schedules. With regard to parental rights, does a parent have the authority to cancel a visit because the child does not want to see the other parent? Is there a threshold at which the parent's rights supersede a court-mandated determination? What about the child's ability to give an autonomous choice concerning visitation, and when does their opinion count? If the visitation schedule is not fulfilled, what are the ramifications and what is the level of tolerance the court is willing to endure? These are only a few questions regarding contact refusal that family courts might encounter with children of divorce.

When dealing with divorce and separation, the relationship between the child and the caregiver becomes vulnerable. There are several theoretical aspects of this relationship that might be taken into consideration. Winnicott's[4] theory of the good-enough mother, John Bowlby's[5] attachment theory between the child and the care-giver, Mahler and colleagues'[6] theory on separation individuation, and Wallerstein and colleagues'[7] extensive work with children of divorce are only a few of the ideas circulating in childhood mental health that help to understand the impact of divorce on children. Not all relationships are created equal, and the parent-child relationship is a prime example. In addition, this relationship is dynamic; it changes over time as the child matures and develops independence. New-onset contact refusal, however, is not a natural progression of this relationship. There is likely a reason for the change, which can range from being completely justified to being irrational and destructive.

Because the relationships of children of divorce involve at least 3 people (the child, the parents, and perhaps other individuals) and their environment, each of these components can be part of the reason for the contact refusal. Although the child is refusing contact, the parents are not irrelevant and their role in the refusal must always be taken into consideration. A parent may unintentionally cause a disruption in the parent-child relationship. This situation is especially true when the parent's coping skills are exhausted and they are experiencing symptoms of depression or anxiety. The parent may not intend to damage the child's interpersonal relationships, but their ability to nurture the child's relationships is simply deficient. Parents also get caught up in the legal process and can lose sight of the children's needs, which creates a form of unintentional emotional neglect that can damage the bond between the child and a parent. Parents who turn to substances are unavailable both emotionally and often physically to the child, which leads to deterioration of the relationship as well.

INTERNAL FACTORS

The child's personality and coping mechanisms can also be held responsible for the relationship problems leading to contact refusal. Children who are stubborn and have an inability to adapt to change are likely to be resistant to the new family structure. Anxious children might succumb to their own worries and be incapacitated, withdrawing into themselves and isolating themselves, leading to contact refusal.

Children may also become angry with their parents for the divorce and the change in lifestyle. Angry children often externalize their problems onto others, such as the targeted parent who the child surmises caused this alteration in their lives. There is also the phenomenon of cognitive dissonance in which children have conflicting emotions for a parent and alter their behavior to alleviate the intolerable affect. There are many other ways in which the child can be the instigator of the contact refusal, but the effect of the environment on the relationship must also be considered.

EXTERNAL FACTORS

Because people and relationships exist in the context of their environment, this too can play an important role in the development of contact refusal. For example, one of the parents typically moves to another home or community, thus creating uncertainty in the child because of the new environment. The child may refuse to see the parent because the new environment is confusing, scary, hostile, or simply unfamiliar. The child may also refuse to see the parent because of other individuals associated with the parent such as a new partner, unfamiliar children in the new household, or perhaps a stranger in charge of supervising the visitation. Occasionally, the custodial parent intentionally causes the child to respond negatively toward the other parent. The custodial parent might be vindictive or attempt to use visitation as a means of leverage. Also, a custodial parent might become dependent on the child and instill a great amount of anxiety such that the child is afraid to leave the custodial parent.

As children mature, their friends become very important figures in their development. Children may begin to identify with their friends more so than their family, and they might push limits and break rules in developing their own identity.[8] This developmental process may lead to contact refusal for a variety of reasons. Adolescents may want to spend time with friends or their significant other or may simply resist as a means of maintaining their own sense of control over their environment. Children and adolescents might also resist visitation because of their access to things they enjoy. These things could include almost anything that children or adolescents feel is important to them, such as a gaming system, their clothes, a pet, or access to a swimming pool. In determining how to respond to the child's contact refusal, it can be helpful to broadly categorize the suspected motive into a pathologic or nonpathologic category.

CLASSIFICATION OF CONTACT REFUSAL

Classification of the child's contact refusal can assist the examiner or health care provider to give recommendations to alleviate the behavior. Classification, however, is not always straightforward. One of the ways to classify contact refusal is to determine if the behavior is pathologic purposeful (PP) or nonpathologic accidental (NPA). The PP category encompasses such phenomenon as child abuse, parental substance use, parental alienation, and purposeful indoctrination. One can see that these destructive phenomena directly affect the parent-child relationship in an unhealthy manner. Abuse can traumatize the child and predispose him or her to future psychological illness. Parental substance use is a form of child neglect. Substance use is also the major cause for separating children from their families and placing them in the custody of the state. The phenomenon of parental alienation is coercive and undermines the parent-child relationship.[9] Purposeful indoctrination is an extreme case in which the child is either overtly or covertly manipulated such that the relationship with the other parent is rejected. These examples are not the only pathologic phenomena that can disrupt the parent-child bond.

Apart from the PP phenomenon, there are also NPA causes that can lead to contact refusal. Nonpathologic causes are not motivated by malice and are often accidental or unintended. Anxiety on the part of the child or the parent, environmental factors, and accidental indoctrination of the child are some examples. Anxiety prevents the child, or custodial parent, from achieving an easy transition to the noncustodial parent. Accidental indoctrination occurs when a parent is unaware that comments made about the other parent influence the child's perception of the other parent. The most obvious nonpathologic reason for contact refusal is the abrupt change in the child's environment. Although going to visit a loved parent, the child has to give up the environment in which he or she is living for a short while. For children, and especially adolescents, peer relationships may be highly important, as well as significant others, their favorite toys, neighborhood activities, and other environment-dependent factors. The child is not only transitioning from parent to parent but also moving to a different environment that may not be as appealing.

Abuse or Neglect of the Child

If the child refuses to visit a parent because that parent was abusive to the child, the child's mother, or some other person close to the child, then contact refusal is normal. Physical evidence of abuse can offer a clear explanation for the resistance, but, as it is known, not all abuse is so overt. In 2008, 16.1% of child maltreatment was because of physical abuse, 7.3% because of psychological maltreatment, and 9.1% because of sexual abuse. The predominant form of maltreatment was child neglect, which accounted for 71.1% of all reported cases.[10] Neglect can largely go unnoticed by persons outside the family and even by the child. Neglect encompasses the child's education, emotional needs, and physical needs. Granted, children may not process educational neglect per se as harmful, but they are likely to understand that a physically or sexually abusive parent is dangerous. Determining the presence or absence of abuse can be a difficult endeavor, but this must be considered as a potential reason for contact refusal.

Case 1

Colby was a 7-year-old boy whose parents recently divorced. They were married for 12 years before his mother filed for divorce because of the father's infidelity in the marriage. After the divorce, Colby had scheduled visitation with his father every other weekend. After about a year, he began to have difficulty transitioning back to his mother's home. He began crying and begging his father not to take him back. Colby told his father that his mother's boyfriend hurt him and that he was afraid of him. Colby's father spoke with his ex-wife about what Colby had said, and she stated that it couldn't be true. She also said that Colby had never approached her about being hurt. During the next visit with his father, Colby had obvious bruises on his back and legs. After his mother could not explain the injuries, an investigation ensued, which revealed that the mother's boyfriend had been teasing and physically abusing Colby.

In this scenario, it is evident that abuse was present, which constituted a perfectly valid reason for the child to resist visitation. Not all cases of abuse are so obvious or so easily determined. Children are often taken from the custody of the parents and placed into state custody until the child's safety has been established.

Some children deny that abuse occurred, when it did, and may even recant an earlier disclosure.[11] The abuse literature gives light as to why children might behave in this manner, but for the purposes here, it is important to acknowledge that if a child denies abuse, it may not be the whole truth. Reasons for recantation of an abuse disclosure include threats made by the abuser to the child, fear of losing contact with a parent or another important figure in the child's life, pressure from the family, judicial proceedings, and perhaps the involvement of protective services.

It is important to consider that the child may be resisting visitation with the parent because of abuse by someone else in the household or community. The child might identify the parent as accepting that behavior and not protecting him or her, thus placing the child at risk for harm. This situation is especially true if the abuser is the parent's new partner (ie, boyfriend). The parent, naive of the abusive relationship, may encourage the child to spend time with that person. There are numerous other possible perpetrators of abuse such as a stepsibling or an individual in the neighborhood or school who bullies the child.

The timing of the contact refusal is important to consider. One might be more likely to suspect abuse if the child was originally visiting the other parent without difficulty and abruptly protests visitation after the parent introduces a new partner to the child. Whenever there is a change in the child's agreeableness to visitation, the parents should look at the psychological, social, and environmental factors that could be causing this new attitude.

When abuse is suspected, it needs to be investigated. If abuse is identified as the cause of the contact refusal, the necessary interventions are straightforward. The child must be safe and the child may need to rebuild a trusting relationship with the parent who allowed abuse to occur. If the parent was the abuser, then this relationship could be considered toxic. Appropriate therapy and supportive measures need to be in place for the child. Rebuilding of the relationship is dependent on the individual circumstances of the case and if the relationship can be healthy.

Purposeful Indoctrination

In some custody cases, parents are involved in a high degree of conflict. The animosity toward the other parent can be so great that the parents use the child as a means of provocation and leverage. Some parents are vengeful and spiteful. When a parent intentionally causes the child to resist visitation with the other parent by way of manipulation and coercing the child's behavior, it is referred to as intentional indoctrination. The motive for the indoctrination is often selfish and does not have the best interests of the child in mind, although parents may believe that they are doing what is ultimately right.

Case 2

Annabel was a 9-year-old girl who was seen crying on the doorstep of her mother's home. A neighbor went over to see if she was all right, and Annabel told her, "My daddy doesn't love me. I hate him." The neighbor, having known the family for many years before the divorce, had seen how Annabel and her father used to play together outside. Annabel continued, "He never comes to visit me after school and my mom says we are going to have to move because he doesn't give us any money. Mom said my daddy found a new family and he doesn't love me anymore." The neighbor overheard Annabel's mother on the phone inside the house. Annabel's mother was yelling at someone, and the neighbor heard her say, "If you don't pay the mortgage, I'll make sure you never see your daughter again!"

In the scenario, it is evident that the custodial parent is malicious in her attempt to cause the child to pull away from the father. The child was told things that were not true, and the parent acted in a way to give those ideas credibility for the child. The child begins to incorporate those new ideas into her conceptualization of the other parent, which negatively influences her attachment. The child begins to alienate the "bad" parent based on falsehoods provided by the "good" parent. This form of contact refusal, which is pathologic and purposeful in nature, may result in parental alienation.

Family therapy is often difficult or even impossible with divorced parents who have a high degree of conflict between them. Mediation is also less likely to produce a compromise, and other forms of legal interventions may be needed. In some cases of parental alienation, reunification therapy, described by Darnall elsewhere in this issue, may be helpful.[12] In some cases, the best treatment for children is to separate them from the unhealthy situation. This separation might mean for the child to stay with another family or enroll in a boarding school. The highly contentious parental relationship is the cause of the contact refusal. As long as the parents continue to involve the child in their dysfunctional relationship, the child suffers.

Accidental Indoctrination

Accidental indoctrination may occur when the parent or someone close to the child exhibits behaviors that influence the way in which the child perceives the other parent. The outcome is unintentional and the indoctrinating parent is usually unaware of the bias that he or she is promoting.

Case 3

Heather was a 6-year-old girl with exercise-induced asthma. Her parents recently divorced, and her mother had primary custody of the child. Before the divorce, Heather had a close relationship with her father. This relationship slowly deteriorated after the divorce to the point that Heather refused to visit her father and clung to her mother during the scheduled exchanges. Beginning when the parents separated, Heather's mother cried at the transition times and repetitively told Heather, "I love you. I miss you. I can't wait for you to come back." During the visitation with the father, the mother called Heather several times a day asking if she was all right and then say, "I miss you so much. I can't wait for you to come home." When Heather returned to her mother, her mother ran to her, became tearful, and said, "I'm so happy you're back. I've been worried sick about you. I don't know what to do when you're gone." The father noticed that Heather began to gravitate away from him. Just before Heather began to refuse visitation with him, she told her father, "Stop being so mean to Mommy. I hate you!"

The scenario depicts an example of unintentional indoctrination of the child against the other parent. Here, the indoctrinating parent is exuding anxiety when the child separates. The parent unknowingly instills doubt in the mind of the child through persistent contact during visitation and emotionally charged transfers between parents. The parent may excessively tell the child that he or she was worried about the child while the child was away with the other parent and may display great relief on returning from the care of the other parent.

Parents with anxiety disorders and dependent personalities might be the most vulnerable to cause accidental indoctrination. For example, the anxious parent causes anxiety in the child that is highest at separation and reunion, which may cause the child to believe that there is reason to doubt the safety of the other parent. Younger children tend to be more sensitive to separation issues and are more vulnerable in situations that harbor intense emotion, which can be both confusing and anxiety provoking.

In addition, dependent parents may parentify the child. Occasionally, a divorced parent may begin to treat the child as an equal. Boundaries are crossed, and the child begins to take on adult responsibilities to meet the needs of the dependent parent. An obvious example is when boys suddenly are thrust into the role of the "man of the house" when the father is away. This parentification may cause the child to bond to the dependent parent out of an inappropriate sense of responsibility and guilt and reject the other parent. This phenomenon is supported through research, which indicates that the socioeconomic status of women decreases after a divorce, whereas that of men tends to increase.[7] Women are left with fewer financial resources and often with custodial care of the children, limiting their employability.

It should be noted that accidental indoctrination does not necessarily have to be caused by the custodial parent. The stepparent, siblings, and extended family can also influence the belief system of the child. For instance, if the maternal grandparents are so angry with their former son-in-law, they may eliminate him completely from their life or begin to speak about him in a negative manner.

Treatment of the relationship between the child and the rejected parent may simply be educating the family and providing guidance. Parents and grandparents may be unaware that their attitudes, comments, and behavior are affecting the child. If this misguiding is identified, the individuals can adjust their behavior or at least help one another keep their behavior in check, especially when around the child. Once the child is no longer exposed to the negative discord, he or she can begin to reestablish a relationship with the alienated parent. Some individuals may apologize to the child for their behavior and work proactively to correct the relationship problems that were created.

Worried Child

An anxious child may exhibit visitation refusal because of an irrational fear that the custodial parent will become unavailable if they separate. The child typically experiences a great deal of sadness, and perhaps guilt, over the separation of the parents. The child has a difficult adjustment to being away from the other parent and interprets this as a loss. This association with sadness and separation of an attachment object reinforces the need to be close to the custodial parent so as to not experience yet another loss.

Case 4

Glenda was an anxious young girl whose parents recently separated. She was scheduled to see her father 2 weekends out of the month. Before the separation, Glenda had a strong attachment to her mother and father. After the separation, Glenda asked her mother, "When is daddy coming home?," to which her mother replied, "Never." Glenda had a significant increase in her anxiety symptoms and began to think that her father was gone forever. Glenda was not comforted by the visitation schedule. She began to develop a sense of abandonment by her father because he was not immediately available. Glenda then began to refuse to leave her mother not only for the scheduled visitation but also for school and other social events. She became fearful that her mother may also abandon her.

The scenario depicts a young girl who experienced her parents' divorce with intense grief and adjustment difficulties. Although her father was alive and well, she lost access to him and felt a sense of abandonment because the mother said he was never coming back. When the time came to separate from the custodial parent for visitation purposes, the child became anxious because of the confusion she had about the visitation schedule. The child was not necessarily refusing contact with the father but was choosing to stay with the custodial parent to avoid the feelings of grief and abandonment. The child had distorted thinking about the relationship she had with her parents and thought that her father had chosen to abandon her. The custodial parent did not play an intentional role in the child's refusal of visitation, although the custodial parent had difficulty reassuring the child.

The worried child needs support and reassurance from both the custodial and noncustodial parents. A child's adjustment problems to the new schedule is not uncommon but should not be prolonged or result in rejection of a parent. If prolongation or rejection occurs, the family may want to consider involving an outside party to assist. Perhaps a guidance counselor at school, a church figure the child trusts, or a family friend might be able to assist. If the child's anxiety continues to be a barrier, the family might want to have him or her evaluated for more specific interventions from a psychologist or psychiatrist. During visitation or at the custodial home, the child may benefit from regular contact with the other parent until the anxiety abates.

Peers and Other Environmental Factors

Children may refuse visitation because of their personal wants and needs and the ability of the noncustodial parent to meet those needs. Children have specific wants and needs in their development, which may supersede their willingness to visit, even with a strong and positive attachment, the noncustodial parent. These wants may dominate their decision making and cause them to refuse visitation.

Case 5

Annah was a 13-year-old girl whose parents divorced when she was 5 years old. Annah had a relatively good relationship with both her parents. The parents had an amicable relationship together, and they both were supportive and active in Annah's life. At age 10 years, Annah began to request different days for visitation and she would occasionally call her father to cancel a visit because of an event with a friend. Her mother and father occasionally agreed to forgo visitation at Annah's request because they knew how important her friends were becoming to her. At age 13 years, Annah had a boyfriend who attended another school but lived in her mother's neighborhood. She refused to visit her father on the weekends to spend time with her boyfriend. She explained, "It's okay 'cause I still see Dad on Wednesday night."

In the vignette, the child placed the desire to be with her friends above the desire to spend time with her father. This scenario is not uncommon, and it is an important consideration when examining the developmental trajectory of a child. One of the developmental tasks of early and middle adolescence is to separate physically and emotionally from parents and to start establishing one's own sense of identity.[8] The child knowingly chooses his or her friends over family and does so regardless of which parent is the noncustodial parent.

Also, children tend to be egocentric and place their desires before the needs of others. Young children, for instance, who want to play with a particular toy or spend time with their pet may be reluctant to leave those things behind to visit with their other parent. This situation might be especially true if the attachment to the parent before the separation was not very strong. Younger children have a difficult time seeing the world from another person's perspective and have difficulty with empathy, so they may not understand the need to visit the other parent and maintain the relationship.

Here, the child continues to have a healthy relationship with the parents, but the environment is the issue. Some children are given their own personal space at both homes (ie, their own room), or the parents might allow them to pack up and take certain items with them between residences. One way to avoid that type of contact refusal is for the child to stay in the same home while the parents come and go. A small number of parents practice nesting in which they move in and out of the child's residence. This approach maintains the child's environment but can become a significant burden on the parents, especially if a parent is dating or remarries. Generally, the parents have to work together to find solutions. The children or adolescents may also have their own ideas of how the custody and visitation arrangements can be altered to meet their needs.

Stubborn Child

Stubborn children experience confusion, discontent, and anger over the separation and divorce of the parents. They do not understand why the parents had to leave each other and do not know how to cope with the change in environment, especially if the change is dramatic. These children, having lost their sense of control of the situation, attempt to regain some of the control by manipulating their parents, both the custodial and noncustodial, through their behavior. For instance, these children may decide to refuse to participate in the parents' divorce by refusing to visit the noncustodial parent, thus negating the separation. The youngster's attempt at control leads to irritation of the parent-child dyad.

Case 6
Brianna was a 12-year-old girl who had a difficult adjustment to her parents' divorce. She lived primarily with her mother and had a typical visitation schedule with her father. Brianna's mother and father occasionally argued on the phone with one another. When it was time for visitation, Brianna told her mother, "Dad can visit me in my room. I'm not going anywhere." She was angry with her parents about the divorce and wanted them to get back together. When Brianna refused visitation, her mother and father would talk on the phone for long periods of time about the visitation schedule and other heated issues about the divorce. Brianna also refused to speak to her father on the phone and told her mother that he can come visit her if he wants to talk.

In this scenario, the child is angry and upset about her parents' divorce and is scrambling for a sense of control and balance in her new family structure. The child is manipulating the parents through her behavior. This type of contact refusal can be solely because of the child's pathology, but, of course, a child's pathology often is partly because of the environment. The adjustment to the divorce has exhausted the child's coping skills, and the parents may not be as vigilant about the child. Parents tend to lose focus of the children's needs during divorce proceedings and can continue to unintentionally ignore their needs postdivorce as well. This situation is especially true in high-conflict divorces and postdivorce relationships that are contentious.[7] In these situations, the parents might be more attentive to the legal matters at hand than the needs of the children. The child is the loser in this case. He or she is experiencing not only a physical separation of parents but also an emotional disruption.

The stubborn child is often angry, and this emotion is usually a barrier for the relationship with the noncustodial parent. Working on uncovering the reason for the anger is an important step in reestablishing the relationship. A stubborn child might also be trying to manipulate the parents in such a way as to bring them back together in a pathologic fashion. In cases of manipulation, it is best if the parents can work together to overcome this behavior.

Child Escaping Conflict

Cognitive dissonance, a well-studied phenomenon of social psychology, is pervasive in situations such as divorce. Cognitive dissonance is an uncomfortable sensation created by the presence of 2 simultaneous conflicting ideas or emotions. The child may love the noncustodial parent but hate that parent because of the divorce and the change in the family structure. To relieve that uncomfortable sensation, which may be experienced as tension, anxiety, or irritation, the child alters his or her attitudes, beliefs, and actions.[13] Dissonance can also be reduced by irrational justification, denial, and externalizing the emotion through blame.

Case 7

Bailey was a 9-year-old boy whose parents divorced several months before a mental health evaluation. Before the divorce, the family saw Bailey as a "chip off the block" because he was very attached to his father. Since the separation, Bailey refused to visit his father. Bailey believed that the divorce happened because his father did something bad. He told the guidance counselor at school that he was mad at his father. Bailey also had more problems sleeping and had not been eating very well. His behavior at school also slightly deteriorated.

The child in this vignette is trying to make sense of the love he has for his father juxtaposed to the confusion and anger he is trying to cope with because of the divorce and adjustment to a new way of life. He sees his father as the reason behind this discomfort. Children, depending on age, have a limited armament of coping skills to deal with such significant changes in their lives. The child may attempt to relieve the dissonance by several means, one of which is attaching to one parent and rejecting the other parent, manifested by contact refusal. Because this action results in disruption of the parent-child relationship, it is referred to as hedonistic dissonance. This specific type of dissonance applies when the adjusting action results in a negative consequence for the individual. In Bailey's case, the disruption of the loving and healthy relationship with his father was damaged rather than improved.

As discussed previously, the amount of postdivorce conflict can have a tremendous impact on this type of contact refusal. If there is high conflict, it is easier for the child to reject the father because it is easier to identify him as the bad guy. If the divorce was mutual and the parents enjoy a low-conflict relationship, then the child might be less apt to blame the father. To reestablish this type of parent-child relational problem, the child should be addressed much like the worried child described earlier. These children need support and reassurance in addition to spending time with the other parent. Allowing the child to skip visitation might enable the idea that the parent is bad. Therapy and guidance is warranted. When the child is present, the parents should not show hostility toward one another because the child incorporates this hostility into his or her irrational thought process.

SUMMARY

Contact refusal is an important concept in both the legal and therapeutic communities when evaluating and treating children of divorce. If this phenomenon is identified, it can be helpful to determine if the cause is pathologic or nonpathologic. This categorization might determine how to intervene, whether it is through a therapeutic process or legal action. The parent-child relationship, as long as it is not toxic, is a critical part of the child's development. It is also important to remember that the parent-child relationship exists within an environment that may have a positive, negative, or neutral effect on the dyad. The child, the parent, and the environment must be considered individually and within the context of one another. The environment refers to not only the physical space surrounding the relationship but also other individuals within the environment. Contact refusal needs to be dealt with and its cause identified because of the importance of the parent-child relationship and to aid in determining appropriate interventions.

REFERENCES

1. Tejada-Vera BSP. Births, marriages, divorces, and deaths: provisional data for 2009. National vital statistics reports, vol. 58. Hyattsville (MD): National Center for Health Statistics; 2010.
2. Amato PR. Children of divorce in the 1990s: an update of the Amato and Keith (1991) meta-analysis. J Fam Psychol 2001;15(3):355–70.
3. Kelly JB. Children's adjustment in conflicted marriage and divorce: a decade review of research. J Am Acad Child Adolesc Psychiatry 2000;39:963–73.
4. Winnicott D. The child, the family, and the outside world. Harmonsdworth (England): Penguin; 1964.
5. Bowlby J. Attachment theory and its therapeutic implications. Adolesc Psychiatry 1978;6:5–33.
6. Mahler MS, Pine F, Bergman A. The psychological birth of the human infant: symbiosis and individuation. New York: Basic Books; 1975.
7. Wallerstein JS, Lewis J, Blakeslee S. The unexpected legacy of divorce: a 25 year landmark study. 1st edition. New York: Hyperion; 2000.
8. Erikson EH. Childhood and society. 2nd edition. New York: Norton; 1963.
9. Bernet W. Parental alienation, DSM-5, and ICD-11. Springfield (IL): Charles C Thomas Pub Ltd; 2010.
10. U.S. Department of Health and Human Services, Administration for Children and Families, Administration on Children, Youth and Families, Children's Bureau. Child Maltreatment 2008. 2010. Available at: http://www.acf.hhs.gov/programs/cb/stats_research/index.htm#can. Accessed February 23, 2011.
11. Ceci SJ, Kulkofsky S, Klemfuss JZ, et al. Unwarranted assumptions about children's testimonial accuracy. Annu Rev Clin Psychol 2007;3:311–28.
12. Darnall D. Beyond divorce casualties: reunifying the alienated family. Lanham (MD): Taylor Trade Publishing; 2010.
13. Festinger L. A theory of cognitive dissonance. Palo Alto (CA): Stanford University Press; 1966.

The Psychosocial Treatment of Parental Alienation

Douglas Darnall, PhD

KEYWORDS

• Divorce • Parental alienation • Psychotherapy

Psychiatrists, mental health workers, and lawyers serving families in court have all heard it before: a mother saying, "He is nothing but a sperm donor," a father trying to contain his rage, saying, "My ex-wife is brainwashing my children with denigrating accusations, so the children are afraid of seeing me because of false allegations of abuse." Observing the hostilities first hand, one can only stand by in frustration thinking how parents can do this to their children and the parent they may have once loved. Most mental health professionals dread the idea of being subpoenaed to court to testify in a custody case. The dread of knowing that the testimony will be challenged makes the professional look like a buffoon before the eyes of the parents and the court. There are also the ethical issues about what can be said in court.[1]

High-conflict parents display a persistent pattern of animosity, hostility, and retribution to each other. Court personnel frequently know the parents by name because of the protracted litigation that appears to have no resolution. The children are dragged along and expected to publicly reject the targeted parent with accusations of abuse, psychological abandonment, or whatever irrational belief the alienating parent can muster. Such behavior promulgates the child's delusional beliefs. The children become the tragic victims of the hostilities. The allocation of parenting time is frequently the parent's battlefield. Parenting time is the spoils of the war.

Over time the true victims, the children, can display serious symptoms of depression, aggressiveness, social withdrawal, and other psychological problems. There is considerable research demonstrating the adverse effects a high-conflict divorce can have on children.[2–4] Wallerstein and colleagues[5] described the impact divorce had on children's lives years later into their adulthood. Although there is some concern about her upper middle class Caucasian sample, she made a dramatic point that high conflict can cause lasting scars. Logic tells us that if children are exposed to a parent's animosity with the intent of depriving them of a loving relationship with

---

Disclosure: The author receives royalties from the publication of books related to this topic, such as *Divorce Casualties: Protecting Your Children from Parental Alienation* and *Beyond Divorce Casualties: Reunifying the Alienated Family*.
PsyCare, Inc, 2980 Belmont Avenue, Youngstown, OH 44505, USA
E-mail address: douglas900@aol.com

the other parent, the consequences for the child later in life can be significant. The children in time will likely suffer from significant emotional distress, the loss of affirmation of knowing they are loved and valued by both parents and the extended family, the void from not having a sense of family continuity, and the loss of potential financial resources.

DEFINITIONS

Parental alienation (PA) is not parental alienation syndrome (PAS). Basically, in this article PA refers to the alienating behaviors of a parent, while PAS refers to the symptoms that are manifested by the child. The first edition of *Divorce Casualties*[6] emphasized the importance of making a distinction between PA and PAS because at the time the book was written, reunification or reversal of severe PA was thought to be near impossible. For that reason, the first edition argued that parents needed to understand the symptoms of PA with the hope of modifying their behavior and preventing the more serious threat to the child, PAS. The distinction is still important for the same reasons, although we can be more hopeful today for successful reunification.

It is also important to understand the difference between PAS and estrangement in this article. In PAS, the child rejects the targeted parent without a good reason or perhaps without any reason at all. In estrangement, the child rejects one of the parents for what the objective observer would call good reason, such as a history of abuse, a mental disorder, substance abuse, or domestic violence.

PARENTAL ALIENATION

Darnall defined PA as "any constellation of behaviors, whether conscious or unconscious, that could evoke a disturbance in the relationship between a child and the other parent."[6(p4)] Typically, one parent is the aggressor and is described as the alienator. The object of the alienation is the targeted or rejected parent. The identity of the alienator is not difficult to determine after ruling out the influences of estrangement. It is important to keep in mind that that alienation is not about "bad guy" versus the targeted parent or "good guy." The roles can alternate between being the alienator and the victim. The targeted parent, feeling victimized, may retaliate with his or her own alienating behavior against the original alienating parent. This process can occur well before PAS appears in the child.

Baker and Darnall[7] conducted an Internet survey of 96 individuals who were self-identified as targeted parents to identify the most frequently reported alienating behaviors. The percentage of the most frequently reported behaviors were:

General badmouthing	74.0%
Creating impression that the targeted parent is dangerous or sick	62.5
Confiding in the child about the court case and child support issues	45.8
Saying the targeted parent doesn't love the child	44.8
Badmouthing targeted parent to authorities	31.3
Limiting visitation	29.2
Confiding in the child about the marriage	29.2
Badmouthing targeted parent's new family or extended family	27.1
Intercepting calls and messages	22.9
Moving away or hiding the child	14.6

Baker and Darnall[7] found that there were no differences between the gender of the targeted parent and gender of the child, meaning that both mothers and fathers were alienating parents and both boys and girls were targets of alienation. However, the gender of the targeted child and the age of the targeted child were associated with the severity of alienation. That is, 55.6% of the targeted girls and 32.6% of the targeted boys were perceived to be severely alienated. Also, targeted children who were perceived as severely alienated were older than the targeted children who were perceived to be mildly alienated. Targeted parents who perceived their children as mild and moderately alienated did not report differences in the number of alienating strategies employed. However, alienating parents identified by the targeted parent as obsessed in their desire to alienate were reported as having more severely alienated children.

PARENTAL ALIENATION SYNDROME

Richard Gardner,[8] the physician who coined the term "parental alienation syndrome," explained that the process was similar to brainwashing except that the motivation for the alienating parent has a conscious as well as "a subconscious or unconscious" component. The children themselves may have motivations that will make the alienation worse. Their hedonistic outlook for immediate gratification or their desire to avoid discomfort makes them vulnerable allies for siding with the alienating parent. Gardner[9(p20)] defined PAS as "...a combination of a programming (brainwashing) parent's indoctrination and the child's own contribution to the vilification of the targeted parent." The child's denigration is unjustified and/or exaggerated. A child's response to a physically or sexually abusive parent is not PAS.

Gardner's[9(p76)] "eight cardinal symptoms of parental alienation syndrome" that focused on the child's behavior included:

- Campaign of denigration, which refers to the child's relentless name-calling, criticizing, and deprecating the targeted parent
- Weak, frivolous, and absurd rationalizations for the child's criticism of the targeted parent
- Lack of ambivalence, in that the child perceives the targeted parent as all-bad with no redeeming qualities and the alienating parent as all-good
- The independent thinker phenomena, which refers to the child's spontaneous insistence that his or her feelings are his or her own, not those of the alienating parent
- Reflexive support of the alienating parent, such that during an argument between the parents, the child will support the alienating parent without any thought or any contemplation that the alienating parent could be wrong
- Absence of guilt over cruelty to or exploitation of the alienated parent, so the child feels no empathy or remorse and, to an outside observer, the child appears to gloat about his or her hate
- Presence of borrowed scenarios, when the hateful child justifies his or her feelings by reciting "memories" or opinions he or she heard from the alienating parent
- Spread of the child's animosity to the extended family of the alienated parent.

Baker and Darnall[10] conducted a second Internet study to examine the relationship between PAS and the 8 symptoms identified by Gardner.[9] The frequencies of PAS symptoms or behaviors reported ("Mostly" or "Always") by 68 alienated parents were:

- Campaign of denigration 87.8%
- Weak, frivolous reasons 98.4%
- Lack of ambivalence 96.9%
- Independent thinking 95.0%

- Express no guilt or remorse 88.9%
- Sides with alienating parent 100%
- Borrowed phrases 79.7%
- Rejects extended family 76.6%.

The study found that the amount of time the child spent with the targeted parent did not prevent PAS. Baker and Darnall[10] said "joint custody is not a *de facto* protective mechanism against PAS." A second finding on a more positive note was that all but one alienated child had something positive to say about the targeted parent, suggesting a window of opportunity for reunification with even the most severely alienated child. All but the one child exhibited some degree of attachment and affection toward the targeted parent.

JUDICIAL INTERVENTIONS

Of course, judges routinely deal with high-conflict divorces and children who are alienated or estranged from one or both parents. In cases of mild PA, judicial intervention alone may resolve the problem. That is, the judge may simply order both parents to support the child's relationship with the other parent and to follow the visitation or parenting time schedule. In cases of moderate PA or PAS, the judge may order a comprehensive treatment approach, usually after hearing the recommendations of a mental health professional. When a court order cannot fix the problems between parents and the children and the judge doubts that the parents can work out their differences, reunification therapy is an option. The features of reunification therapy are discussed later in this article. In cases of severe PA or PAS, when the alienating parent and the child have adopted intractable false beliefs about the targeted parent, there are no simple answers or interventions for resolving the impasse. Proposed solutions range from doing nothing and hoping the problem will go away to making an involuntary change of custody to the alienated parent. That possibility is also discussed later in this article.

Judicial decisions are ordinarily based on the "best interests of the child," which is a complex notion. It is more than simply identifying which parent will foster a loving relationship between the children and the other parent. Alienated parents do not understand this. For the alienated parent, being a target of alienation is a good enough reason for him or her to gain custody. Frequently attorneys fail to educate their client about other factors involved in making a custody order. The alienated parent must keep in mind that a parent's refusal to foster a loving relationship with the rejected parent is only one of many criteria for deciding best interest. The alienated parent needs to know all the criteria concerned with a court's decision, especially issues that involve estrangement.

Angry parents enter the court ready to attack, and expect to defend their arguments in typical adversarial manner. The parent may think his or her story is unique, believing that the judge cannot help but agree with the parent's arguments. However, the judge has heard the stories many times over and may have little interest in which parent is right and who is wrong. Blaming does not help the children. The court focuses on making a decision that appears fair, lessens the conflict between the parties, and ultimately protects the children.

The judge will assess arguments in light of how the local jurisdiction defines the child's "best interests." The judge may agree that alienation has occurred, but place less weight on that argument than on other criteria. For example, if a parent has been convicted of domestic violence, the judge will put more weight on the history of abuse than alienation.

Judges have the right to use their discretion on how they weigh the various factors defining best interests. Some states have no written criteria defining "best interests," so the judge uses his or her experience to decide what is best for the child.

REUNIFICATION THERAPY
Definitions

There is a distinction between what is referred to as reunification and reunification therapy. Reunification emphasizes case management, making use of court-appointed mediators, parenting coordinators, or special masters to monitor compliance with court orders and educate the parents about working together.[11,12] Reunification therapy, on the other hand, is a recently developed therapeutic modality for treating high-conflict, litigious families.[3,12–15] Reunification therapy occurs between the therapist and the family. The focus is threefold: tempering the hostilities of the alienating parent; assuring an emotional and safe environment for the children with both parents and significant others; and repairing the damaged relationships with the children. The term "reunification therapy" is becoming more common, although there are few detailed treatment protocols for this form of treatment.

Although these approaches are effective for most high-conflict families, they are less effective with the severely alienated child and the obsessed parent. Reunification alone does not address the unique problems with these parents and children who refuse any cooperation with the targeted parent. Reunification therapy remains a difficult task because the alienating parent and child usually have little or no desire to participate in the therapy, and may try to sabotage any gains made with the children, miss appointments, and discount any value from the therapy. This can be a good argument for removing the children from the alienating parent if he or she persists with this pattern of behavior during the reunification process.

The Reunification Team

Reunification is brought about by a team of professionals identified by the court: a guardian *ad litem*, a parenting coordinator, visitation center staff, a reunification therapist, and anyone else that the court believes should be involved. The court usually decides the composition of the team with the agreement of parents' attorneys. Successful reunification involves a team of qualified specialists, each with a specific responsibility. Preparing for reunification is a challenging process. There is more to the preparation than obtaining a court order and telling the parents that they must participate in the process.

Role of the Therapist

The reunification therapist must have the flexibility to work with all parties and freely exchange information among them. The therapist cannot have an allegiance to one parent or child to the detriment of the others. Before initiating reunification therapy, the therapist will ask the parents to sign an informed consent form that explains the therapy guidelines, grant a waiver of confidentiality, and assign responsibility for fees. There can be no protection of confidentiality between the parents, children, judge, or other court-appointed persons. All of the parties must understand this before the start of the reunification therapy. Protecting a parent's past medical or mental health records is the exception; those records remain confidential.

The reunification therapist should not be expected to testify or to make custody or visitation recommendations. That aspect of the therapist's role should be understood by all before a therapist is assigned to the family. Testifying and making custody or visitation recommendations is considered unethical because of the prohibition against dual relationships. Some treatment approaches may include both a reunification therapist and a parenting coordinator. Whereas the reunification therapist would not make recommendations to the court regarding custody or visitation, the parenting coordinator may make such recommendations. For example, the parenting coordinator may testify that one parent has completely cooperated with the treatment plan whereas the other parent has been very uncooperative with the plan, and the coordinator might conclude and recommend that the former parent be given custody or greater access to the children.

Focus on the Parents, Not the Child

A judge looking into the faces of the hostile parents and a child refusing parenting time or visits with the targeted parent will frequently order the child into therapy. Such an approach to reunification rarely works, for good reason. Children forced into counseling rarely like counseling. They will complain that counseling is boring and that it interferes with other more desirable activities such as playing with their friends. Children will typically blame the targeted parent for being forced into counseling, which adds to the divisiveness rather than facilitating reunification. There are additional ramifications for the children. The child becomes the identified patient, suggesting that the problems between the parents are his or her fault. Equally devastating to the children is the implication that they are responsible for repairing the damage between the parents.

The child should never be the primary focus of reunification therapy. The parents, not the child, should be ordered to participate in reunification therapy. The parents, not the child, have the power to change. If there is to be a change in the child's anger and distorted thinking, the parents together must learn how their irrational beliefs are harmful to the child.

Role of the Child

Although the child is not the primary identified patient, the reunification therapist must have court approval to access the child for occasional meetings. The therapist monitors the child's attitudes and behaviors as a way to measure the progress of the parents' treatment. Also, the therapist may use those meetings to help the child achieve a more realistic view of the targeted parent and to lessen the child's anxiety against the targeted parent. Children who have been victims of PA need the opportunity to build a new history with the targeted parent, while the targeted parent is coached on how to rebuild the relationship with the children without getting defensive or attacking. Frequently parents ask, "what should I do with the children in a particular situation?" The answer is to do or say whatever will reduce the child's anxiety.

Sometimes, therapy for the child is appropriate when there is significant deterioration in the child's global functioning. The reasons may have nothing to do with alienation. If the reunification therapist finds the child's general functioning is impaired for whatever reason, a different therapist may need to intervene. Impaired functioning may be manifested by a drop in school grades, signs of depression, impaired social relationships, or belligerent behavior outside the context of the divorce. If the child already sees a therapist, he or she should continue. The child's therapist should know that the family is participating in reunification therapy.

Considering the Child's Preferences

The child should not feel caught in the middle; children should never have to choose one parent over the other. That principle supports the argument for not having laws allowing a child to elect custody or choose a custodial parent. Child advocates may argue that children should have the right to choose, but for the alienated child the consequences are too severe because the child's judgment is questionable. The child's public pronouncement of choosing a parent becomes the ultimate rejection, and is difficult for the child to take back. For these reasons, many states have eliminated the age of election, meaning the age a child is able to choose where to live. Instead, most states have a provision for the child to express his or her wishes, but the decision still rests with the court and what is considered to be in the child's best interest.

Reunification is not choosing the rejected parent over the alienating one. However, both parents must respect the child's dignity and right to have a reciprocal relationship with both parents, free of interference and exposure to further alienating or estranging behaviors from either parent.

The Alienating Parent

Alienating parents are more likely to comply with court orders if they know their behavior and compliance to court orders are monitored. Parents obsessed with their desire to alienate may ignore court orders, believing that no one is going to tell them what to do. These parents believe they must protect the children at all costs, arguing that the court does not understand the risks involved with the child having a relationship with the rejected parent. Courts expect those parents to explain the reasons for their refusal to cooperate, so the parent may have to defend the reasons why he or she should not be sanctioned.

Parents risk sanctions if the court believes the parent's arguments are irrational or unfounded. The court may give a parent a second chance, and targeted parents are angered when they see the alienating parent getting only a "slap on the hand" for noncompliance. Unfortunately, after a couple of slaps on the hand the alienating parent's arrogance and defiance are reinforced. The following case illustrates the way one court set limits on an alienating parent.

Case 1

Emma, though the custodial parent of her 3 girls, was frustrated and hurt because she had not seen her daughters for 5 months because they refused to return from their father's home after an extended summer visit. The father of the girls expressed contempt toward the court to the extent that he went to jail twice for 10 days each because he refused to comply with court orders about the financial settlement. He argued before the court that Emma was a risk to the children's safety because she was "emotionally unstable," though he could not give any rationale to support his beliefs. The girls wanted nothing to do with their mother, believing she could harm them. The girls refused to talk with her on the phone, avoided eye contact while waiting in the hallway for the court hearing, and expressed relentless anger.

The court found no evidence presented by the father or the children that Emma was a threat to their safety. The court concluded that this was the "worst case of parental alienation" that had come before the court and ordered the immediate return of the children to the mother. The court ordered reunification therapy and forbade the father from having any contact with the children until the court proceedings 4 months later were completed. The judge said that the only "damage he saw was the danger created" by the father himself. The judge also ordered that if the court found that the father willfully and wantonly violated the court orders, father would serve "30 days in jail for each count of the five (5) contempt charges to be served consecutively for a total of one-hundred and fifty (150) days."

Both parties agreed on a reunification therapist. The therapy began with identifying the realities that both parents and children must accept: the court orders; the fact that continued litigation and alienation harms the children; state laws supporting both parents' involvement with the children; and that neither parent is going to disappear. Facing these realities, both parents must assume personal responsibility for how they behave and learn to readjust their beliefs and behavior. Failing to do so runs the risk that the court will impose serious sanctions, which could include a change of custody.

Forcing or coercing an alienating parent with threats if they do not change his or her behavior may work for a short time, but not for the long term. Lasting change will only occur when there is a change in the parent's belief system or behavior.[14] In private moments the alienating parent will frequently express the opinion that the rejected parent should just disappear, making life easier for everyone (Darnall DC. The content validity of parental alienation. Unpublished raw data, 1993).

The Targeted Parent

Sometimes the targeted parent can be the greatest obstacle to successful reunification. In the following vignette, Robert's anger and belief that the court betrayed him is a good example.

Case 2

Robert had custody of his two sons, ages 7 and 11, since the divorce. His wife Christina filed for custody when she heard the boys complaining about their father's anger. The court ordered a custody evaluation, which described in detail the children's complaints about their father's anger. The children were willing to continue seeing their father but wanted to live with their mother. Robert was ordered by the court to enroll in an anger management class. The order was humiliating to Robert because he vehemently denied the allegations. After 3 years had passed, the allegations continued. The court ordered an updated custody evaluation because there were 9 criminal complaints filed and investigations conducted by the Department of Human Services for child abuse against the father. The psychologist who conducted the custody evaluation was clearly frustrated about what had occurred during the past 3 years with the children, and father's failure to get treatment for his anger. The psychologist recommended that all contact between Robert and the children be terminated. The recommendation enraged Robert. For months he had not seen his children and saw little hope of reunification. Later, all complaints against the father were dismissed.

Robert was surprised to receive an e-mail from his attorney saying that Christina was willing to ignore the psychologist's recommendations and consider reunification. Robert was cautiously optimistic and sought help to better understand how reunification works. During the discussions, Robert's anger and insistence that the children know the lies that had been perpetuated about him tended to derail the process. He wanted someone to acknowledge the lies told by the children and the psychologist. He wanted to be righted for all the wrongs that he felt inflicted on him. Contrary to what his attorney said to Robert, he could not shake the injustice that he felt. Robert's anger was understandable, but his failure to control his passion hurt him and his cause. A challenge for many targeted parents is learning to control the intensity of their emotions. Some of these parents are not very likeable by the time they go to court. Robert may not have appreciated how his anger was feeding into his ex-wife's argument that he was volatile and abusive.

The Extended Family

A new significant other or a grandparent can destroy any progress parents and children make in their therapy. The alienating parent's source of support (spouse and extended family) may need to participate in the therapy and be educated about their contribution to the problem. The reunification therapist must have the ability to interview and educate anyone that may play a role in the alienation.

All Family Members Must Accept Change

The reunification therapist's task is to identify the realities that both parents must live, that is, the probability of that any further alienating behavior will harm the children.[16–19] State laws and courts support the children's right to have a reciprocal loving relationship with both parents. Both parents must reconcile themselves to those realities by changing their behavior, and most importantly their beliefs about what is best for the children.

Reunification therapy can be time consuming because the alienation may have been going on for a long time and the alienating parent will frequently resist change. The alienating parent must learn to empathize with what the children are feeling, put self-serving interests aside, and reframe his or her beliefs. Targeted parents must learn how to rebuild their relationship with the children and avoid their own alienating behavior. The children will have to learn to differentiate reality from their delusional thinking. Children learn that they can have an opinion about either parent, but their opinion should be founded on personal experience rather than what they are told by an angry or hurting parent.

ACCESS TO THE CHILD

If a parent is prevented from spending time with his or her children, the parent has no chance of preventing further damage from alienation or repairing the damaged relationship. Having access to the children is imperative. The targeted parent's attorney must advocate for his or her client to have continued parenting time with minimal supervision. Allegations of abuse or threats to the children's safety are the only good reasons for severely restricting parenting time or requiring supervised visits. The parent must abide with supervised visits rather than lose all time with the children. The angry parent must be told by the attorney to swallow his or her pride and comply with the court-ordered supervised visits. The parent stands a better chance of continuing or rebuilding a relationship with the children if he or she complies with the court order.

SUPERVISED VISITATION

Courts will order supervised visits when there is a concern about the children's emotional or physical safety, or have reasons to believe that the children are afraid of the rejected parent. Sometimes the court's decision for supervised visits is attributable to false information provided by the alienating parent. The risk of ordering supervised visits is the subtle message to the child that the targeted parent is a threat to the child's safety. The threat can be reinforced by the alienating parent's comments, such as, "Honey, don't worry, the nice lady at the center will protect you."

Supervised visits should only occur in conjunction with reunification therapy or a court-ordered intervention to repair the damaged relationship. Supervised visits alone simply mean that the court has designated someone to observe the parent and children during limited visits. Supervised visits will limit how a parent can interact with his or her child. Visits are usually limited to one room or the center's backyard. Physical affection, leaving the center for a fun activity, or sharing a relaxed day at home is discouraged or not allowed. Restricted access helps ensure the child's safety but limits the parent's ability to heal the relationship. Because of the center's rules, both the parent and the child feel inhibited. The rules may restrict hugging or exchanging gifts. A theory behind supervised visits is to give the parent additional time to regain the child's trust and feel more comfortable together.

Older children may feel bored during the supervised visit, later complaining that "I don't want to go back to the center." When the older child complains, the alienating parent may use the child's compliant to support the argument that the child wants nothing to do with the targeted parent, rather than blaming the child's attitude on the restricted environment. The person supervising and observing the visits should report any progress or problems during visits to the court.

Case 3

The alienating parent may look for reasons to argue that supervised visits are a failure and should be discontinued. An example is the mother who was told that her son warmed to his father, and together had a great time. In response, the mother grabbed her son's hand and ran out of the visitation center, never to be seen again. This mother was not interested in her son's having an affectionate or fun relationship with his father. The mother's agenda was clearly more important than what was best for her son.

COURT ORDERS

Ideally, court orders that mandate supervised visits should address important practical questions such as:

- What criteria should the visitation center or guardian *ad litem* use to extend or eliminate supervised visits? The criteria should be an improvement in the parent-child relationship rather than a calendar date.
- What reparative or corrective actions should be taken by the staff of the visitation center to promote an improved parent-child relationship?

Ideally, the court order should distinguish the role of the reunification therapist from the role of the parenting coordinator. In particular, the court should not assign arbitration responsibilities, such as the authority to modify parenting time, to the therapist. In many states, doing so is unethical and places the therapist in an awkward position of being the gatekeeper. The therapist who functions as an arbitrator becomes the object of the parents' manipulations, which detracts from the therapy or places the therapist in a position to defend the decision to reduce or increase parenting time.

On the other hand, a parenting coordinator may function as an arbitrator and have the authority to modify parenting time. A parenting coordinator is an impartial individual assigned by the court to monitor progress, make certain limited decisions, and offer recommendations to the court to modify access. The parenting coordinator should usually consult with the reunification therapist before making significant decisions. The family will save considerable time and money if the court grants the parenting coordinator limited arbitration power to make quicker decisions and changes in the parenting time schedule.

IMPASSES AND STALEMATES

It is not uncommon for the reunification therapist to encounter bumps, potholes, and road blocks. For example, the alienating parent may avoid meeting with the therapist or communicating with the targeted parent. The therapist cannot be expected to track down an uncooperative parent; that is not the therapist's responsibility. If one of the parents refuses to cooperate, the therapist should notify the court, parenting coordinator, or the referral source, usually one of the attorneys or the guardian *ad litem*. Sometimes the cooperating parent will need reassurance from his or her attorney that the alienating parent's failure to comply will hurt the offending parent in court, providing the court has the reputation of not tolerating blatant failure to follow court orders. Emma's case, discussed earlier, can attest to this. Both parents must believe there are sanctions for failing to follow court orders.

During the course of reunification the parents or the child may encounter a crisis that could stifle reunification. The crisis does not have to be a bump in the road, but can be an important opportunity that may motivate a change in the parents' behavior. There are anecdotal reports that a crisis will prompt an oppositional parent to cooperate with court orders and allow the targeted parent to resume parenting time. Dealing with the crisis should occur in the context of the reunification therapy.

Crises may occur because of a variety of life events. However, there are also ways by which the court can create a crisis that may reduce an uncooperative parent's resistance to change. A crisis can arise from circumstances in the parent's life or from a court's intervention. The judge in Emma's case is an example of the court's creating a crisis. The court and the professionals involved in the case must be vigilant in looking for an opportunity to create a suitable crisis. A crisis can take many forms, such as the following.

The Stalemate that Hurts

A stalemate usually refers to a situation in a game in which neither player can win. Divorcing parents may find themselves in a no-win situation, when they realize that continuing to fight for their position harms not only themselves but most importantly the child.

A Recent Catastrophe

Sometimes a shared crisis will bring people who have been fighting for years together. Science fiction movies have made use of this theme in the films *War of the Worlds* and, more recently, *Independence Day*. Both plots involved aliens who threatened the existence of the earth, so the nations of the world united against a common enemy.

Impending Catastrophe or Deteriorating Position

Both parents are more likely to break their stalemate when they can see and agree that any inaction on their part will lead to a crisis that will hurt their child. For example, failure to obtain emergency medical treatment can have devastating effects on their child's health.

An Enticing Opportunity

An opportunity may arise with a child that demands the parents' cooperation or their working together. Taking advantage of this type of crisis requires the parents to think about what is best for the child rather than their own narcissistic needs. There are many possible enticing opportunities, such as: completing the college financial statements for scholarships; graduation from high school, college, or even graduate school; extensive medical treatment; and an important family event, including weddings and funerals.

A Judicial Crisis

Rather than waiting for a crisis to develop, the court may want to consider creating its own crisis for the warring parents. A judge can create a crisis to motivate the unmotivated parent. Frequently the court will limit its intervention to a lecture with a well-meaning threat to sanction the uncooperative parent. When deciding how to intervene, the court has to decide between doing nothing and hoping the problem will go away, or creating a crisis.

For example, a judge might threaten to put the children in foster care, which gives the parents reasons for putting their differences aside. The judge creates the circumstances for motivating the parents and extended family to change because the crisis now has more to do with the children than the parents' need to control. In one such case, the parents and extended family were in a hurting stalemate because they and their children were in a no-win situation unless they cooperated. When they were threatened with foster care, the parents and the children shared the potential of an impending catastrophe, and without a shared solution each were placed in a deteriorating position. To avoid the crisis, the court provided an enticing opportunity for these parents by offering the pathway to resolution through mediation and reunification therapy.

If the court chooses this approach, the crisis and the consequences of the crisis should affect both parents and not harm the child. The court may consider the following methods to create a crisis.

- Considering a change of custody to the targeted parent. The alienating parent needs to understand the possibility of the change of custody before going to court.
- Transferring the children's temporary custody to a responsible family member.
- Ordering one or both parents to sit in the county jail long enough to understand the consequences for failing to comply with court orders. This has been done, with positive results.
- Requiring the alienating parent to put a significant sum of money in an escrow account to pay for missed appointments and court expenses that the compliant parent may incur for returning to court.
- Filing criminal charges for contempt and then allowing for a plea bargain to include cooperation with court orders.
- Granting extra parenting time for the targeted parent to make up for times that the alienating parent failed to provide the child for visitation.

For the crisis to work, the court cannot bluff. The court must follow through with the threat and realize that the court and the targeted parent will be the target of the alienating parent's rage. In many jurisdictions, the parents do not take the court's threats seriously. The court will lose credibility in the eyes of both parents if the noncompliant parent only receives a slap on the hand. Therefore, the alienating parent must be sincerely frightened by the order. He or she must believe and feel the crisis. However, there must be an escape clause in the court order that generally involves both parents. The escape clause specifically describes to both parents what is expected to avoid the consequences of their contempt. Finally, the court—not the targeted parent—must be responsible for the court's decision. This fact must be emphasized to the alienating parent and the children. The judge should invite the children into the courtroom and explain to the children the court order, and emphasize to the children that it is the court and not either parent that is making the order and that they are expected to comply with the court order.

PRACTICAL CONSIDERATIONS

There are many obstacles to reunification, a serious one being the cost. Reunification therapy can take months of intense work with the parents. Insurance companies will frequently refuse to pay for court-ordered therapy because insurance is intended for treating mental disorders and not relationship problems (V-codes). Even if the

DSM-5 (*Diagnostic and Statistical Manual of Mental Disorders*, Fifth Edition; in development) accepts PA disorder as a diagnosis, it will not guarantee insurance reimbursement because the disorder will likely be viewed as a relational problem and not a mental disorder. Parents will likely carry the financial burden for the treatment. Another concern that few attorneys consider when making a referral for therapy is that the insurance companies require a valid mental health diagnosis for payment. The diagnosis can later be used in court, suggesting that the parent either has a serious mental disorder or the therapist is fraudulently claiming a mental disorder so he or she can get paid. A wise therapist will never take this risk, knowing they could later have to defend the diagnosis in court.

SPONTANEOUS REUNIFICATION

When all hope for reunification is lost, there are circumstances when the alienated child or "adult child" will reach out to the targeted parent. Darnall and Steinberg[20,21] sought to understand how and why these children/adults reached out to their alienated parent. Together they identified 27 severely alienated children and found that each child/adult had something in common with each other. Each child/adult reached out in response to a crisis in his or her life, believing that somehow the alienated parent might be helpful. The wise parent was comfortable with knowing he or she was being used or taken advantage of, but was willing, hoping that he or she might reestablish a meaningful relationship with the son or daughter. The reunification came about without mental health counseling or court intervention. The study by Darnall and Steinberg offers hope for alienated parents who believe they have forever lost their children.

CRITERIA FOR SUCCESSFUL REUNIFICATION

Successful reunification can be judged from different perspectives. The criteria for successful reunification are different for the alienated child, the alienating parent, and targeted parent, and the court. The court's goals for successful reunification may include: the parents' never returning to court; the parents' facilitating a reciprocal loving relationship between the children, the parents, and extended family; and repair of any damage done to the child's relationship with the alienated parent. For the alienated child, successful reunification is to feel safe and trust that both parents will attend to their basic emotional and physical needs. Children do not want to be exposed to their parents' hostilities or petty arguments. The child wants to feel and express affection toward both parents without emotional repercussions. For the targeted parent, the goals are to reduce alienating behavior, strengthen his or her relationship with the child while reducing conflict with the other parent, and repair the damage that alienation has caused the child. The targeted parent's goal is to enjoy unimpeded parenting time with the child and heal the suffering caused by previous alienation. The goal for the obsessed parent is typically the total removal of the targeted parent from the child's life. That goal is contrary to successful reunification therapy. If the criteria for successful reunification are to include the child's opportunity for a reciprocal positive relationship with both parents, the outcome studies must include verification from both parents.

POSSIBILITY OF FAILED REUNIFICATION

Successful reunification implies more than a successful reconnection between a rejected parent and the alienated child. Reunification must include the child's having a reciprocal and safe relationship with both parents. Some mental health professionals may disagree because of the concern that the alienating parent is emotionally abusive and manipulative, arguing that a more realistic goal involves helping the child reconnect with the targeted parent and undoing the negative programming by the alienating parent. Adopting this alternative goal implies that the alienating parent may not change, which can certainly be true. Success may include limited contact with the alienating parent.

There may be concern about who should define the criteria for denying an alienating parent access to his or her child and under what circumstances such should occur. Assuming that the child's safety is not an issue, the decision to deny access should be made after sincere attempts to reunify have failed and the likelihood of continued alienation persists. It is especially important to consider denying the alienating parent access to the child when there continues to be false allegations of abuse. Also, persistent noncompliance with court orders represents failure of reunification, and may result in denying the alienating parent access to the child.

CONSIDERING CHANGE OF CUSTODY

The difficulty the court has before changing custody is deciding, on balance, what is best for the child: maintaining the status quo, knowing that the child is making an adequate adjustment, or taking a risk in changing custody. Changing custody is thought to be very risky for most judges, especially with the severely alienated child who vehemently expresses a hatred or fear of the rejected parent. The court may freeze with its own fear when it hears that the child will run away or kill himself or herself if they have to spend time with the targeted parent, while the other side is yelling about fairness and his or her right to have a loving relationship with the child. Making a decision under such circumstances can be extremely stressful. Courts have looked to mental health professionals for guidance. Unfortunately, there are few outcome studies supporting either position's impact on the child's global adjustment. This area of research is one that needs to be addressed, but there are serious problems with this type of study because of an insufficient sample size and identifying a treatment and control group.

Gardner[22] advocated an involuntary change of custody or forced visitation in cases of severe PAS. He conducted a follow-up study of 99 children from 52 families, that is, cases that he had personally consulted on. For 22 children, the court followed Gardner's recommendation to reduce the alienating parent's access to the children or transfer custody to the targeted parent. Subsequently, the PAS symptoms of all of these 22 children were reduced or eliminated. For 77 children, the court did not follow Gardner's recommendation to reduce the alienating parent's access to the children or transfer custody to the target parent. Subsequently, the PAS symptoms of 7 of the 77 children were reduced or eliminated although they remained with the alienating parent, while the PAS symptoms of 70 of the 77 children were not reduced or eliminated. There were limitations to Gardner's study, which involved follow-up interviews with the targeted parent but not the alienating parent. He reasoned, probably accurately, that the alienating parent would not want to talk with him or provide accurate information about the child's adjustment with the change. The conclusion of the study, while taking into consideration the limitations, is that an involuntary change of custody is a viable option for reducing or eliminating PAS. Not known is the quality of the relationship between the children and the alienating parent when a change of custody occurred.

CONSIDERING PREVENTION

The worst phrase for a parent to hear is "I don't want to see you ever again. I will run away or kill myself." After hearing the contempt in the child's voice and recovering from the shock of disbelief, the parents and the court can be frozen with fear. No one can shake the child back to reality. Despite all the discussion of PAS in recent years, there are still no validated treatment protocols for reversing the damage caused by the overly zealous parent. There continues to be speculation about the effectiveness of changing the alienated child's custody to the targeted parent. Then, there is the misguided notion of simply referring the child for therapy, frequently reinforcing in the child's mind that he or she is at fault, or at least that he or she is responsible for maneuvering his or her life between two warring parents. It is easy to see that such a recommendation rarely works.

Preventing PAS is much easier that treating a family damaged by a severe degree of alienation. There is a need for courts and attorneys to identify local resources offering parents educational programs or parenting classes that teach parents how to prevent alienation and how to focus on building and keeping strong the relationship between the parents and children. If such a program does not exist in a community, the court may suggest to the local mental health center that it develops such a program.

SUMMARY

Reunification therapy is a complex process that requires a therapist to be experienced not only in that specialized form of treatment but also in family therapy and cognitive behavioral therapy. The goal of reunification therapy is to assist the parents to change not just their behavior but also their destructive beliefs. The parent may use false beliefs to rationalize his or her alienating behavior, such as "I am only trying to protect my children," when no evidence of abuse exists.

During the course of reunification therapy, parents must accept the following realities: that both parents agree that continued and protracted litigation harms children; that state laws support the value of children having a reciprocal, loving relationship with both parents; that it is important to obey court orders; and finally, the reality that neither parent is going to disappear from their children's lives.

Reunification therapy requires active collaboration between the therapist, the court, and other agents, such as the parenting coordinator. Through its authority, the court can greatly support the reunification therapist, providing the parents fear the sanctions that will be imposed by the court for noncompliance to the court orders. The children will be the beneficiaries of this teamwork between the court and the therapist.

REFERENCES

1. American Psychological Association. Guidelines for child custody evaluations in family law proceedings. Am Psychol 2010;65:863–7.
2. Amato PR. Children's adjustment to divorce: theories, hypothesis, and empirical support. J Marriage Fam 1993;55:23–38.
3. Barris MA, Coats CA, Duvall BB, et al. Working with high-conflict families of divorce: a guide for professionals. Northvale (NJ): Jason Aronson, Inc.; 2001.
4. Wallerstein JS, Kelly JB. Surviving the breakup: how children and parents cope with divorce. New York: Basic Books; 1980.
5. Wallerstein JS, Lewis J, Blakeslee S. Second chances: men, women and parents cope with divorce. New York: Mariner; 2001.
6. Darnall DC. Divorce casualties: protecting your children from parental alienation. Dallas (TX): Taylor Publishing Company; 1998.
7. Baker AJ, Darnall D. Behaviors and strategies employed in parental alienation: a survey of parental experiences. J Divorce & Remarriage 2006;45(1/2):97–124.
8. Gardner RA. Recent trends in divorce and custody litigation. Academy Forum. A Publication of the American Academy of Psychoanalysis 1985;29(2):3–7.

9. Gardner RA. Parental alienation syndrome. 2nd edition. Cresskill (NJ): Creative Therapeutics; 1998.

10. Baker AJ, Darnall D. A construct study of the eight symptoms of severe parental alienation syndrome: a survey of parental experiences. J Divorce & Remarriage 2007;47(1/2):55–76.

11. Sullivan MJ, Kelly JB. Legal and psychological management of cases with an alienated child. Fam Court Rev 2001;39(3):299–315.

12. Ellis E. Divorce wars: interventions with families in conflict. Washington, DC: American Psychological Association; 2000.

13. Darnall DC. Beyond divorce casualties: reunifying the alienated family. Dallas (TX): Taylor Publishing Company; 2010.

14. Johnston JR, Walters MG, Friedlander S. Therapeutic work with alienated children and their families. Fam Court Rev 2001;39(3):316–33.

15. Lampel A. Post-divorce therapy with high-conflict families. Indep Pract 1986;6(3): 22–6.

16. Baker AJ. Adult children of parental alienation syndrome: breaking the ties that bind. New York: W.W. Norton; 2007.

17. Hodges W, Bloom B. Parent's report of children's adjustment to marital separation: a longitudinal study. J Divorce 1984;8(1):33–50.

18. Long N, Forehand R, Fauber R, et al. Self-perceived and independently observed competence of young adolescents as a function of parental marital conflict and recent divorce. J Abnorm Child Psychol 1987;15(1):15–27.

19. Johnston J, Kline M, Tschann J. Ongoing post-divorce conflict: effects on children of joint custody and frequent access. Am J Orthopsychiatry 1989;59(4):576–92.

20. Darnall DC, Steinberg BF. Motivational models for spontaneous reunification with the alienated child: part I. Am J Fam Ther 2008;36(2):107–15.

21. Darnall DC, Steinberg BF. Motivational models for spontaneous reunification with the alienated child: part II. Am J Fam Ther 2008;36(3):253–61.

22. Gardner RA. Should courts order PAS children to visit/reside with the alienated parent? A follow-up study. Am J Forensic Psychol 2001;19(3):61–106.

Visitation Arrangements for Impaired Parents

Stephen A. Montgomery, MD*, David F. Street, MD

KEYWORDS

- Impaired parent • Visitation • Forensic mental health
- Substance abuse

A common question posed to mental health professionals by the legal system is whether the visitation rights of parents with significant mental illness should be restricted in any way because of their condition. Much like psychiatric and psychological parenting and custody evaluations, there is little empirical research to answer such questions. This article describes a suggested methodology for providing useful clinical information to the court to help guide their decisions in these complicated matters. The research on the impact of various mental disorders on parenting abilities is briefly reviewed. Case vignettes will be provided to illustrate how these impairments present to the forensic examiner.

Parents may be impaired by a variety of mental disorders. Historically, parents with more severe chronic conditions, such as schizophrenia, bipolar I disorder, substance dependence, and mental retardation, have been severely limited in their visitation rights with their children. However, it is now widely recognized, at least in the literature, that the critical factor is not merely the presence of a specific diagnosis but the impact that condition has on parenting abilities. Perhaps the only diagnoses that would automatically preclude safe parenting would be untreated pedophilia and severe mental retardation.

Several researchers have studied the impact of a variety of mental disorders on parenting abilities in both animal and human subjects. Although those studies do shed some light on how certain mental disorders may affect parenting abilities, such research is typically not focused on answering specific legal questions, such as visitation parameters for mentally ill parents. Because knowledge of that body of research may aid forensic evaluators in forming their final opinions, the research findings across 4 broad categories of mental impairments are briefly reviewed.

SUBSTANCE ABUSE

Substance abuse may have a negative impact on parenting skills in a variety of ways. The obvious acute effects of intoxication from most substances of abuse will impair

The authors have nothing to disclose.
Department of Psychiatry, Vanderbilt University School of Medicine, 1601 23rd Avenue South, Nashville, TN 37212, USA
* Corresponding author.
E-mail address: stephen.a.montgomery@vanderbilt.edu

Child Adolesc Psychiatric Clin N Am 20 (2011) 495–503
doi:10.1016/j.chc.2011.03.009
1056-4993/11/$ – see front matter © 2011 Elsevier Inc. All rights reserved.

childpsych.theclinics.com

judgment, impulse control, alertness, concentration, decision making, and contact with reality. All these domains are critical for adequate parenting of children. Secondary effects include the negative influence on occupational and financial capacities of the parent, increased risk for other criminal activities, time demands in obtaining and using the substance that detract from the time with the children, and the more chronic effects of both active use and withdrawal states on the parent's mood.

A recent study of 45 parents with serious mental illness found that severe substance abuse was the only factor that correlated with less frequent parent-child contact during the 30-month study period.[1] Neither psychiatric diagnosis nor severity of psychiatric symptoms was a significant factor in predicting parent-child contact when substance abuse was taken into account. Substance abuse has also been determined to diminish parental supervision. Several studies suggest that children whose mothers abuse alcohol or other drugs are at increased risk for physical, academic, and socioemotional problems.[2,3]

Case 1

Ms X was a 32-year-old woman who was court ordered to undergo a comprehensive psychiatric parenting evaluation. Ms X had a long psychiatric history including several inpatient hospitalizations. For several months, she was totally disabled from working because of her psychiatric conditions. She suffered from a variety of psychiatric conditions, including alcohol dependence, bipolar disorder, posttraumatic stress disorder, and a personality disorder with cluster B features. Her outpatient treatment had been provided by her primary care physician and included some medications with the potential for abuse, such as benzodiazepines, pain medications, and muscle relaxants.

Concerning behaviors were a fractious relationship with her husband and his family as evidenced by intense verbal arguments and acrimonious electronic messages. Police intervention had been required on multiple occasions because of Ms X's behavior. Several months before being evaluated, Ms X spent 45 days in jail for a second DUI conviction. She also reported drinking a few beers to help sleep while her infant napped. Staff at her supervised visitations had to remind her repeatedly of the rules of the visitation facility.

Information provided to the court included complete *Diagnostic and Statistical Manual of Mental Disorders* (Fourth Edition, Text Revision) psychiatric diagnoses with detailed explanations of each diagnosis, a summary of all her past psychiatric treatments, and a summary of all the concerning incidents with her child and spouse. Recommendations for assessing and improving the stability of her multiple conditions were provided. The recommendations included remaining out of the hospital, transferring outpatient care to mental health specialists (as her primary care provider had already recommended numerous times), remaining abstinent from alcohol, eliminating all prescription medications with the potential for abuse, cessation of volatile arguments and communications with her husband and his family, and refraining from further incidents of dyscontrol requiring police intervention. In the meantime, her parenting time was supervised.

PSYCHOTIC DISORDERS

Active psychotic symptoms that directly incorporate the children are obviously concerning. Delusions that the child is possessed, has special powers, is medically sick, or must be sacrificed are rare but potentially disastrous.[4] A study of 39 severely mentally ill mothers found not guilty, by reason of insanity, for killing their children found that 69% of the mothers were experiencing auditory hallucinations at the time of the offense.[5]

Psychotic disorders can present other issues. Some parents with schizophrenia have difficulty reading and responding to subtle nonverbal cues, which are essential for adequate parenting.[6] Women with schizophrenia show the least engagement with their infants, followed by women with mania, and then women with depression.[7] Some studies have shown that women with schizophrenia have poor prognosis for improving in their parenting skills even after recovery from acute episodes especially if they are single mothers with little social support to assist with caregiving.[8,9] A comparison of severely mentally ill women divided into 2 groups, 1 who were caregivers for children and 1 without such duties, revealed a significantly greater proportion of psychotic diagnoses in the non-caregiver group. The caregiver group had more affective diagnoses.[10]

Case 2
Mr Y was a 36-year-old man referred by his attorney for an evaluation to assist with his regaining custody of his son. He related a 6-year history of psychiatric treatment of bipolar disorder. He had never been hospitalized. He was currently not receiving any mental health outpatient treatment but continued to be prescribed 2 anti-seizure medications by the Health Department to treat his neuropathy and bipolar disorder. His child had been removed by the Department of Children's Services (DCS) because of concerns about his living conditions: lack of heat, lack of water, and inadequate clothing for the child. DCS was also concerned that Mr Y was stalking various state caseworkers and evaluators.

On examination, Mr Y was hypomanic. He spoke about a variety of conspiracy theories. When queried about his child, he gave appropriate and detailed responses regarding the child's abilities, daily schedule, and needs. Similarly, he gave appropriate responses regarding various hypothetical parenting situations involving children of varying ages, based on the Parenting Assessment Skills Survey.

In conclusion, Mr Y seemed to have a significant mood disorder best characterized as bipolar II disorder. His condition was not fully stable. His mood state was mildly hypomanic. He still endorsed mild quasi-delusions, that is, nonbizarre beliefs that were probably shared by a small subset of the general population. Mr Y had not incorporated his child into any of these delusions. His parenting skills seemed intact. Once the issue of proper environmental conditions was addressed, the main barrier to resuming custody was removed. Psychiatric treatment was recommended but not an absolute condition for resumption of visitation rights.

MOOD DISORDERS

Depressed mothers are more likely to stop breastfeeding and report difficulties managing their infants' crying and demands.[8,11] Depressed mothers are more self-absorbed and more apt to miss infant cues and thus seem withdrawn and disengaged.[8] Highly depressed mothers seem to have a more profound impact on children than schizophrenic mothers.[10] Although filicide is a rare occurrence, psychiatrists may underestimate the prevalence of filicidal thoughts. One study found that more than 40% of depressed mothers with children younger than 3 years endorsed thoughts to harm them.[12]

PERSONALITY DISORDERS

By definition, individuals with personality disorders have impairments in at least 2 of the following areas: cognition (ie, ways of perceiving and interpreting self, other people, and events); affectivity (ie, the range, intensity, lability, and appropriateness of emotional response); interpersonal functioning; and impulse control.[13] Substantial impairments in any of these domains can potentially compromise parenting skills.

A prime example is borderline personality disorder, which has been viewed by some as a model of disturbed parenting.[14] Borderline personality disorder has been associated with an increased incidence of disorganized attachment behaviors and ongoing interactional difficulties between parent and child.[15] Specific abnormalities of fronto-limbic regulatory systems that have been demonstrated in neuroimaging studies of borderline personality disorder seem to correlate well with deficits in normal parenting skills, such as attachment, reading and responding to infant cues, stress tolerance, and emotional regulation.[14]

Case 3

Mr Z was a 21-year-old man court ordered to undergo a psychiatric evaluation after refusing to comply with transferring his child back to the mother, the custodial parent, after his visitation. Mr Z knew that others were aware of his longstanding difficulty with mild obsessive-compulsive disorder (OCD). He feared that this label would be used to deny him continued visitation with his child.

Interview and history did indeed confirm a diagnosis of OCD but also revealed significant symptoms consistent with generalized anxiety disorder and a situational type specific phobia of driving. More significant were Mr Z's behaviors that led to the referral in the first place, including his inability to cooperate with exchanges with his ex-girlfriend and mother of his child, regressive behaviors, and anxiously clutching the child and crying hysterically when it was time to transfer the child to the mother. His communications with his ex-girlfriend vacillated among desperate pleas to reunite, scorching devaluation of her character, and wishes for her to have nothing to do with the child. In these communications also, Mr Z threatened to kill himself and the child. Thus, a provisional diagnosis of borderline personality disorder was made.

Mr Z had no history of psychotic symptoms, inpatient treatment, substance abuse, or criminal arrests. He was receiving psychiatric medication management from a psychiatric nurse practitioner. He had supportive parents, but they too were unable to convince him to be more reasonable and compliant with the visitation transfer process.

In analyzing this case, Mr Z's psychiatric conditions had direct impact on his parenting because they interfered with visitation with the mother and involved direct threats to harm himself and the child. Although his overall risk for following through on these threats was rated as low, such threats could not be ignored. The diagnosis of mild OCD did not seem to interfere with his parenting abilities and was not a significant factor in the final analysis.

The evaluator recommended that Mr Z receive more specialized mental health treatment with a psychiatrist and an individual psychotherapist. His stability would then be measured by his progress or lack of progress regarding the following: compliance with the recommended treatments; lack of need for inpatient psychiatric hospitalization; lack of inappropriate communications electronically or otherwise with his ex-girlfriend or his family; and lack of inappropriate behaviors during visitation exchanges and during visits with his child. As Mr Z progressed in those areas, gradually increasing levels of visitation and custody arrangements were recommended.

EVALUATING THE IMPAIRED PARENT

This article narrowly focuses on addressing the impact of parental mental illness on visitation arrangements. The authors understand that in many parenting or custody evaluations, this impact will only represent a small aspect of a comprehensive evaluation, which may include evaluations of both parents and all involved children.

The method of evaluating a potentially impaired parent follows the same general guidelines as with any forensic psychiatric evaluation. A comprehensive psychiatric history and examination should be performed to include the typical areas, such as history of the present illness, past psychiatric history, substance use history, past medical history, current medications, family and developmental history, educational history, marital and relationship history, occupational history, social history, financial history, legal history, and the children's history.

It is important to assess the parent's knowledge of the needs of children of the same age as those of the evaluee, which would include awareness of their child's milestones and capabilities, daily needs and schedules, and other factors specific to their children. The significance of a parent's particular impairments will most likely vary depending on the child's developmental phase. A detailed account from the parent regarding the current issues with custody and visitation that have resulted in the referral should also be obtained.

An important step in the parenting evaluation, as with most forensic evaluations, is to obtain and review as many collateral sources of data as possible, which should include any legal documents related to the proceedings, such as motions filed by either party, court transcripts, court orders, and police reports. The person's official criminal history record should be obtained and reviewed. Any documents from the DCS should be reviewed. As many past psychiatric treatment records as possible should be obtained. Also, any documentation of correspondence between the parents via e-mail, text messages, or postings on social network sites should be obtained. Other family members may be helpful in providing ancillary information regarding past family history, the person's history of mental illness, and their current functioning.

Although traditional psychological tests have not been extensively studied for their use in measuring the dimensions valuable in parenting, they still may be a useful adjunctive measure to the evaluation. Typically, testing is most useful in helping to assess how forthcoming and open the parent is in providing information about his or her mental illness. Therefore, tests such as the Minnesota Multiphasic Personality Inventory-2 and the Personality Assessment Instrument, which contain validity measures that can provide information about the person's symptom management style and defensiveness, are most useful. Tests specifically designed to detect malingering, such as the Structured Interview of Reported Symptoms, are usually not helpful, because the person being evaluated is highly motivated to appear as psychologically healthy as possible, as opposed to exaggerating, magnifying, or outright faking symptoms of mental illness.

Specific tests for parental capacities may be useful. One example is the Parenting Awareness Skill Survey, developed by Bricklin and colleagues,[16] which asks the parent to describe how they would manage several brief scenarios involving children of a variety of ages.

ANALYZING THE DATA
Is Mental Illness Present?

Sometimes, persons are referred for forensic evaluations because both parents agree to be evaluated even though only 1 of them has a history of mental illness. Thus, some parents will simply not have a significant mental disorder. Alternatively, a parent may have a mental disorder, but the symptoms are in full remission.

Does the Mental Illness Compromise Parenting?

This is the critical question that must be addressed. No specific test will answer this question. The clinician must infer this causal relationship from the parent's history, observations of the parent's interactional skills during the interview, observations and/or reports of the parenting style with their children, and ancillary sources of data about parenting skills.

The areas to consider for parenting include the knowledge of the child and age-appropriate needs; degree of contact with reality and whether specific psychotic symptoms incorporate the child directly; impulse control; ability to be properly attuned and responsive to the child's needs; problem-solving skills; and interpersonal skills for both direct interaction with the child and other important individuals in the child's life. Whenever possible, such impairments should be supported by specific examples of problematic behaviors from the parent's history rather than global statements such as "Persons with disorder X lack parenting skill Y." Caution must be exercised by the clinician in rating this domain because mental health professionals tend to impose a higher minimum standard of adequate parenting than the legal system recognizes.

Is the Mental Illness Stable?

Issues important to assess stability include responsiveness to medication and other treatments, compliance with medication and other treatments, and the natural history of the mental illness. The course can vary from the chronic waxing and waning of schizophrenia, the phasic nature of bipolar disorder, or the static nature of mental retardation.

Stability can be assessed in several ways. One measure is frequency of hospitalization. If the person's mental disorder is so unstable that he or she requires inpatient treatment every few months, his or her condition is most likely not stable enough for independent visitation. Another measure is treatment compliance. If a person routinely misses mental health treatment appointments and takes his or her medications inconsistently, he or she is at greater risk for relapse and recurrence of the illness. Reviewing treatment records of the impaired parent is helpful in determining stability. If the records designate the patient's condition as in remission with high Global Assessment of Function scores and decreasing frequency of visits, then this typically correlates with greater stability.

How Can the Mental Illness Best Be Stabilized?

Recommendations for appropriate mental health treatment should be provided. Stipulations should specify that the person is compliant with all recommended treatments, which may include psychotropic medication, therapy visits, and abstinence from substance abuse. Medication levels may be useful for compliance, and random drug screens may be used to establish remission of substance abuse. Other recommendations may include appropriate communications with the other parent and their family members; no legal involvement such as police being called to the home; and, of course, no allegations of child abuse or maltreatment.

What Compensatory Factors Are Present?

Gauging the strength of the impaired parent's support network is helpful. The presence of a supportive family and friends who can assist the impaired parent not only with the demands of childrearing but also with monitoring and assisting in treating the person's mental illness cannot be overemphasized. The parent's insight and compliance with the treatment should be evaluated. One study found that better insight into their mental illness was associated with more sensitive mothering and lowered assessed clinical risk of maltreatment.[17] Insight has been shown to be a predictor of better illness outcomes,[18] better treatment compliance,[19,20] and better occupational and psychosocial functioning.[21]

TYPICAL RECOMMENDATIONS
Develop a Formal Support Network

A formal support network comprises individuals who know the parent, such as the other parent, therapist, psychiatrist, coworker, friend, relative, neighbor, new spouse, and so forth. A list should be prepared with every person's name and contact information. The impaired parent signs the list and agrees that everyone in the network can communicate with one another whenever anyone has any concerns about the impaired parent's condition. One person should assume a leadership role for the network. That person should be given the authority to interrupt or suspend the impaired parent's parenting time until it can be addressed by the court. That role would typically be appropriate for the parenting coordinator if there is one involved in the case.

Having such a formal support network will prevent scenarios in which a person later explains, "I didn't have permission to notify anyone that the parent was becoming psychotic and delusional, so it's not my fault that he abducted his baby." The formal support network should be reassuring to the custodial parent who may worry about the child when in the care of the impaired parent.

Provide a Plan for Progression of Visitation

After making an accurate psychiatric diagnosis, the evaluator should provide the court with useful information regarding the parent's current and future functional abilities. Parents who are acutely psychotic or manic or actively abusing substances are usually deemed unstable and unfit for unsupervised visitation. Conclusions in those cases are usually fairly straightforward. The more difficult determinations are when the person has been stabilized, perhaps after a recent hospitalization.

How long of a period of stability is necessary before the person can resume independent parenting? Again, the time frame depends on the nature and severity of the person's mental illness and how the illness directly affects their parenting skills. As a general rule, parents with severe mental disorders should remain out of the hospital for at least 1 year before considering them psychologically stable, in full remission, and able to have full unsupervised visitation.

Generally, the first criterion an individual needs to meet to resume visitation is that they can safely be in a professionally supervised environment with the child. Subsequent responsibilities and privileges should be increased in a gradual stepwise manner. As the parent-child interactions are monitored and appropriate behaviors are observed, the time allowed should be increased. The next step would be supervised visits at home with supervision by another relative or responsible adult. Then, they can progress to independent day visits and then overnight visitation.

SUMMARY

Many challenges remain regarding the assessment of visitation and parenting privileges. Current models of parenting that come from the child development and child maltreatment fields are too narrow in their focus to act as a foundation for such evaluations and are often based on research with select groups in the society, making them open to bias.[22] Race, ethnicity, and socioeconomic status have been shown to affect parental diagnosis and play a major role in the processes of parenting.

Yet, mental health professionals are still in the best position to evaluate mentally ill parents and provide useful information to the courts regarding visitation privileges. Although little research has been conducted to directly answer that specific legal question, staying informed of the general research about mental illness and parenting abilities will assist the forensic examiner with the task.

The literature makes it clear that mental illness is likely to be only a small part of the total risks parents experience, which include family disruptions and conflicts, single-parent status, social isolation, and financial and other stresses associated with living in poverty.[23] Similarly, the contribution of the mental health professional, although valuable, is usually only a small portion of a more complex legal analysis. Therefore, mental health professionals provide education and recommendations, but ultimately these questions are answered by the legal system.

REFERENCES

1. Jones D, Macias R, Gold P, et al. When parents with severe mental illness lose contact with the children: are psychiatric symptoms or substance use to blame? J Loss Trauma 2008;13(4):261–87.
2. Smith M. Parental mental health: disruptions to parenting and outcomes for children. Child Fam Soc Work 2004;9:3–11.
3. Conners NA, Bradley RH, Mansell LW, et al. Children of mothers with serious substance abuse problems: an accumulation of risks. Am J Drug Alcohol Abuse 2004;30(1):85–100.
4. Kumar R, Marks M, Platz C, et al. Clinical audit of a psychiatric mother and baby unit: characteristics of 100 consecutive admissions. J Affect Disord 1995;33: 11–22.
5. Friedman SH, Hrouda DR, Holden CE, et al. Child murder committed by severely mentally ill mothers: an examination of mothers found not guilty by reason of insanity. J Forensic Sci 2005;50(6):1466–71.
6. Persson-Blennow I, Naeslund B, McNeil TJ, et al. Offspring of women with nonorganic psychosis: mother-infant interaction at one year of age. Acta Psychiatr Scand 1986;73:207–13.
7. Riordan D, Appleby L, Faragher B. Mother-infant interaction in post-partum women with schizophrenia and affective disorders. Psychol Med 1999;29:991–5.
8. Murray L, Cooper P, Hipwell A. Mental health of parents caring for infants. Arch Womens Ment Health 2003;6(2):71–7.
9. Appleby L, Dickens C. Mothering skills of women with mental illness. BMJ 1993; 306:348–9.
10. White C, Nicholson J, Fisher W, et al. Mothers with severe mental illness caring for children. J Nerv Ment Dis 1995;183:398–403.
11. Seeley S, Murray L, Cooper PJ. The detection and treatment of postnatal depression by health visitors. Health Visit 1996;64:135–8.
12. Jennings KD, Ross S, Popper S, et al. Thoughts of harming infants in depressed and non-depressed mothers. J Affect Disord 1999;54:21–8.
13. American Psychiatric Association. Diagnostic and statistical manual of mental disorders. Text revision. 4th edition. Washington, DC: American Psychiatric Association; 2000.
14. Newman LK, Harris M, Allen J. Neurobiological basis of parenting disturbance. Aust N Z J Psychiatry 2011;45(2):109–22.

15. Newman LK, Stevenson CS, Bergman LR, et al. Borderline personality disorder, mother-infant interaction and parenting perceptions: preliminary findings. Aust N Z J Psychiatry 2007;41:598–605.
16. Bricklin B, Elliot G, Halbert M. The parent awareness skills survey (PASS). In: Bricklin B, editor. The custody evaluation handbook: research-based solutions and applications. New York: Brunner/Mazel Publishers; 1995. p. 88–91.
17. Mullick M, Miller L, Jacobsen T. Insight into mental illness and child maltreatment risk among mothers with major psychiatric disorders. Psychiatr Serv 2001;52: 488–92.
18. McEvoy JP, Appelbaum PS, Geller JL, et al. Why must some schizophrenic patients be involuntarily committed? The role of insight. Compr Psychiatry 1989;30:13–7.
19. Amador XF, Strauss DH, Yale SA, et al. The assessment of insight in psychosis. Am J Psychiatry 1993;150:873–9.
20. Lysaker P, Bell M, Milstein R, et al. Insight and psychological treatment compliance in schizophrenia. Psychiatry 1994;57:307–15.
21. Soskis DA, Bowers MB. The schizophrenic experience. J Nerv Ment Dis 1969; 149(6):443–9.
22. Azar S, Lauretti A, Loding B. The evaluation of parental fitness in termination of parental rights cases: a functional-contextual perspective. Clin Child Fam Psychol Rev 1998;1(2):77–100.
23. Oyserman D, Mowbray C, Meares P, et al. Parenting among mothers with a serious mental illness. Am J Orthopsychiatry 2000;70(3):296–315.

Estimating Present and Future Damages Following Child Maltreatment

David L. Corwin, MD[a,b,*], Brooks R. Keeshin, MD[c]

KEYWORDS

- Child abuse • Child maltreatment • Damage
- Forensic evaluation

Nearly half a century has passed since Henry C. Kempe and his colleagues published their vanguard article describing the "battered child syndrome."[1] Three decades have passed since child sexual abuse reemerged into public and professional awareness[2] after 2 previous cycles of discovery and suppression over the last 150 years.[3] Billions of public dollars have been spent and continue to be spent on efforts to protect children from child maltreatment through child welfare agencies, law enforcement, courts, foster care, prevention, research, and health care. These efforts are based in part on the evidence provided by thousands of publications and studies addressing various aspects of child maltreatment identification, investigation, treatment, and prevention.

Along with the emergence of child maltreatment as a major focus of public and professional attention has come the realization that in some cases there are parties who have legal responsibility and financial assets. Civil liability for the harms associated with child maltreatment creates a demand for child psychiatrists and other mental health professionals with forensic expertise to provide estimates of the present and future damages following child maltreatment. This article seeks to assist professionals involved in personal injury child maltreatment cases where the central question is damage caused by the maltreatment. It briefly reviews current knowledge about the present and long-term harms of child maltreatment, and suggests an approach for

The authors have nothing to disclose.
^a Pediatrics' Child Protection and Family Health Division, University of Utah School of Medicine, Salt Lake City, UT, USA
^b Primary Children's Center for Safe and Healthy Families, 675 East 500 South, Suite 300, Salt Lake City, UT 84102, USA
^c Child Abuse Pediatrics, Mayerson Center for Safe and Healthy Families, Cincinnati Children's Hospital Medical Center, 3333 Burnet Avenue, Cincinnati, OH 45229, USA
* Corresponding author. Primary Children's Center for Safe and Healthy Families, 675 East 500 South, Suite 300, Salt Lake City, UT 84102.
E-mail address: david.corwin@imail.org

Child Adolesc Psychiatric Clin N Am 20 (2011) 505–518
doi:10.1016/j.chc.2011.03.005
1056-4993/11/$ – see front matter © 2011 Elsevier Inc. All rights reserved.

evaluating and formulating expert opinions regarding the damage and recommended treatments to ameliorate these harms throughout the lives of child maltreatment victims. The article does not address many other possible questions that may arise in this kind of litigation including liability, standard of care, or apportioning harm among multiple sources of trauma.

PHYSICAL INJURIES

Children who are physically or sexually abused are reported to experience several illnesses and disabilities directly related to tissue damage or exposure during the abuse. Bruises, burns, and fractures sustained during abuse can have acute pain and potentially long-term disability.[4] Traumatic brain injury, as seen in the abusive head trauma of infants and young children (formerly known as the cranial manifestations of shaken baby syndrome), have well-documented neurological deficits in cognition, speech, sensory, motor, as well as potential mood and behavioral changes.[5,6] Overall lifetime costs associated with individuals who have suffered severe traumatic brain injury have been estimated at over 4 million dollars.[7] In sexual abuse, genital injuries may result in acute pain and increase the risk for long-lasting effects such as sexual dysfunction, urinary problems, sexually transmitted infections such as human immunodeficiency virus, and reproductive problems.[4,8]

Along with injury and disability directly related to tissue damage during maltreatment, certain diseases are more often present among individuals with a history of abuse. This correlation has been observed in such populations as those who suffer from obesity, irritable bowel syndrome, fibromyalgia, and other chronic pain conditions.[9–12] Subsequent studies have shown a generally increased risk of poor health and use of the medical system among individuals with a history of childhood maltreatment.[13]

PSYCHOLOGICAL AND BEHAVIORAL SEQUELAE

There are several problems that occur more often among sexually abused children than in nonabused children.[14] Although some child victims of sexual abuse display few initial effects, the majority show some signs of posttraumatic stress,[15] and more than one-third meet diagnostic criteria for posttraumatic stress disorder (PTSD).[16] Increased anxiety, fears, emotional lability, depression, oppositional and conduct disorders, and substance abuse are other reported sequelae to sexual abuse.[17–19] Interpersonal difficulties, increased rates of revictimization later in life, and increased risk for suicide are encountered more frequently among child sexual abuse victims than in other children and adolescents.[20,21] Alterations in cognition, perceptions, and beliefs including increased guilt and shame are also more prevalent in the wake of child sexual abuse.[22,23] Although many of these problems are shared with victims of other forms of child maltreatment, alterations in sexual knowledge, emotional reactivity, and behavior are more specific to experiences of child sexual abuse.[17,24] Recent advances in brain imaging and biological research suggest that child maltreatment negatively influences brain development.[25–27] Symptoms of attention-deficit/hyperactivity disorder and dissociative disorder are also found among both sexually abused and physically abused children more often than among nonmaltreated children.[28]

The effects of physical abuse on children are similar to sexual abuse,[29] with one-third meeting criteria for PTSD[30] and, in one study, 81% having some posttraumatic stress symptoms.[31] Physically abused children also have more aggressive and noncompliant behavior problems as well as more depression than nonabused children.[32]

PSYCHOLOGICAL MALTREATMENT

Psychological maltreatment and neglect are associated with many serious short-term and long-term problems, and are intrinsic to all forms of child maltreatment.[33] Hart and Brassard[34] define psychological maltreatment to include spurning, terrorizing, isolating, exploiting/corrupting, denying emotional responsiveness, and mental health, medical, and educational neglect. Affective and cognitive problems noted among victims of psychological maltreatment include increased anxiety, depression, immaturity, suicidal ideation, lowered self-esteem, negative thinking styles and views, and emotional instability.[35] Victims are at increased risk for social and behavioral problems including substance abuse, eating disorders, impulsivity, antisocial behavior, attachment problems, diminished empathy, dependency, sexual behavior problems, aggression, juvenile delinquency, and adult criminality.[36] Learning difficulties, lower measured intelligence, increased academic problems, and lower achievement are also more common.[37] Long-term health problems including allergies, asthma, hypertension, somatic complaints, increased rates of infant mortality, and physical and developmental delays are more frequent in this population.[38]

FUTURE HARMS OF CHILD MALTREATMENT

The Adverse Childhood Experiences Study is the first large study to examine the association between childhood adversities and the likelihood of suffering from common illnesses of adulthood.[39] The adverse childhood experiences include direct victimization (physical, sexual, or emotional abuse), witnessed victimization (domestic violence), or other markers of household dysfunction (illicit substance use by family, family mental illness, or family who were incarcerated). The first wave of the survey reviewed responses of more than 9500 members of Kaiser Permanente in California. The initial analysis of the study found that as an individual's number of adverse childhood experiences increased, so too did the likelihood of smoking, drug abuse, or alcoholism, with a 2- to 12-fold increase in risk among those with 4 or more adverse childhood experiences.[39] Furthermore, among individuals with multiple adverse childhood experiences, there was a significant increase in the risk of suffering from common adult diseases such as depression, cardiovascular disease, cancer, and lung and liver disease.[39] Strengths of the study include that it is a large, population-based study that covers a variety of adverse childhood experiences rather than just focusing on one form of abuse. Limitations of the study are that it is cross-sectional, counts all experiences equally when analyzing the data, and relies solely on historical recollection of childhood adversities, which may result in underreporting of childhood adversity. It also addresses a population covered by private health insurance, which is probably healthier and more functional than the general population.

Wegman and Stetler[40] performed a meta-analysis on 24 articles that examined adult medical outcomes among individuals who had suffered from childhood physical and/or sexual abuse. Effect sizes, as opposed to odds ratios, were reported in the analysis so that studies that used both dichotomous and continuous variables could be included. By convention, effect sizes of 0.2 are considered small, effect sizes of 0.8 or more are considered large (with no upper limit), and effect sizes of 0.5 are considered medium.[41] The analysis demonstrated that the effect size for child abuse on overall health outcomes as an adult was 0.42 (95% confidence interval 0.39–0.45), indicating a small to medium effect. Large effect sizes were demonstrated for musculoskeletal and neurological problems (reported effect sizes of 0.94 and 0.81, respectively). Similar correlations have been demonstrated in other large-scale studies that have examined medical outcomes among individuals with a history of abuse (**Table 1**).[42–44]

Table 1
Selected large population-based studies and meta-analyses reporting the correlation between childhood maltreatment and adult physical and mental illness

Study	Type	Population	Childhood Experience	Adult Medical Correlation	Adult Psychiatric Correlation
Felitti et al,[39] 1998	Cross-sectional community survey	>9500 adult members of Kaiser Health Plan in 1995–1996	Adverse childhood experiences (ACE)[a]	Odds Ratios[b]: >3 ACEs: Heart disease 2.2 Cancer 1.90 Stroke 2.4 Severe lung disease 3.9 Severe obesity 1.6	Odds Ratios[b]: >3 ACEs: Suicide attempt 12.2 Depressed mood 4.6 Alcoholism 7.4 Illicit drug use 4.7 Intravenous drug use 10.3
Molnar et al,[50] 2001	Cross-sectional community survey	>5800 adults in 1990–1992 National Comorbidity Survey	Childhood sexual abuse	—	Odds Ratios[b]: Females: Depression 1.9 Posttraumatic stress disorder (PTSD) 10.2 Severe drug dependence 1.9 Any mental illness 2.3 Males: PTSD 5.3 Any mental illness 2.3
Springer et al,[43] 2007	Longitudinal population-based cohort	>2000 middle-aged adults in the Wisconsin Longitudinal Study last interviewed in 1994	Childhood physical abuse	Odds Ratios[b]: Arthritis 1.34 Asthma 1.64 Bronchitis/Emphysema 1.49 Hypertension 1.43 Ulcer 1.84	Odds Ratios[b]: Anxiety 1.78 Depression 1.61 Anger 2.02

Study	Design	Sample	Exposure	Cohen d Effect Sizes[c] / Other	Odds Ratios[b] / Other
Fergusson et al,[52] 2008	Longitudinal population-based cohort	>1000 adults followed until age 25 in New Zealand	Childhood physical and sexual abuse	—	*Odds Ratios*[b]: Childhood sexual abuse: Mental illness 2.4 Childhood physical abuse: Mental Illness 1.5
Wegman and Stetler,[40] 2009	Meta-analysis	24 studies	Childhood physical and sexual abuse	*Cohen d Effect Sizes*[c]: Poor health 0.42 Cardiovascular 0.66 Respiratory 0.71 Gastrointestinal 0.63 Neurological 0.81 Musculoskeletal 0.94	—
Green et al,[54] 2010	Cross-sectional community survey	>5600 adults in 2001–2003 National Comorbidity Survey	Childhood adversity: Maltreatment Interpersonal loss Parental maladjustment	—	*Population Attributable Risk Proportions*[d]: Mood 26.2% Anxiety 32.4% Substance use 21% Disruptive behavior 41.2%
Dube et al,[42] 2010	Cross-sectional community survey	>5300 adults in the Texas Behavioral Risk Factor Surveillance System Survey of 2002	Adverse childhood experiences (ACE)[a]	*Odds Ratios*[b]: Any childhood abuse: Obesity 1.5 Fair or poor health 1.7 Childhood abuse *and* Household dysfunction: Obesity 1.3 Fair or poor health 2.0	—

(continued on next page)

Table 1
(continued)

Study	Type	Population	Childhood Experience	Adult Medical Correlation	Adult Psychiatric Correlation
Irish et al,[44] 2010	Meta-analysis	31 studies	Childhood sexual abuse	*Odds Ratios*[b]: General health problems 1.48 Gastrointestinal symptoms 2.12 Gynecologic symptoms 1.90 Pain 1.65 Cardiopulmonary symptoms 1.36 Obesity 1.73	—
Chen et al,[51] 2010	Meta-analysis of longitudinal studies	37 studies	Childhood sexual abuse	—	*Odds Ratios*[b]: Anxiety 3.09 Depression 2.72 PTSD 2.34 Suicide attempts 4.14

[a] Adverse childhood experiences include 3 abusive experiences (physical, sexual, or psychological abuse) and 4 types of household dysfunctions (domestic violence, family drug use, family mental illness, or incarceration) retrospectively reported.

[b] Odds Ratio: measure of strength of association between 2 variables, where Odds Ratio of 1 is a random occurrence, and the higher the Odds Ratio, the greater the association (ie, Odds Ratio of 2.0 indicates that the association observed is twice as likely as would be expected by chance alone).

[c] Cohen d Effect Size: by convention, an effect size of 0.2 is considered small, 0.8 is considered large, and a medium effect size is between the 2 extremes (approximately 0.5).

[d] Population Attributable Risk Proportions: percent of risk of the development of the disorder that is attributable to the correlated condition.

Similar to the evolution of research regarding observed correlations between childhood maltreatment and long-term adverse health effects, there is a considerable amount of literature that supports the correlation between maltreatment and child and adult mental illness. Although PTSD is commonly thought of in association with abuse,[45] different studies have demonstrated significant correlations between abuse and the occurrence and manifestation of anxiety disorders,[46] mood disorders such as depression,[47] bipolar disorder,[48] and psychosis[49] in adults. Again, criticism of some initial research in this field is that the populations studied are primarily clinical, whereby the participants are already more likely to suffer from mental illness and there is concern that this information may not reflect the general population. Population-based studies, meta-analyses, and studies that include a variety of childhood adversities attempt to address the previous concerns of potential bias only when looking at the correlation of childhood maltreatment and mental illness.

Molnar and colleagues[50] interviewed more than 5000 individuals in a representative sample and inquired about history of childhood sexual abuse, and past and current psychiatric illness. In the sample, 13.5% of women and 2.5% of men reported a history of childhood sexual abuse, which was limited to repeated fondling and attempted or completed rape before the age of 18 years. When those who reported childhood sexual abuse are compared with those who did not report childhood sexual abuse, there are statistically significant increases in mood, anxiety, and substance use disorders among women, and PTSD and substance use disorders among men. When all of the disorders are collapsed, 78% of women and 82.2% of men who reported a history of childhood sexual abuse reported at least one psychiatric disorder, compared with 48.9% of women and 51.1% of men who denied a history of childhood sexual abuse.

A meta-analysis of longitudinally based studies with comparison groups examined the correlation between sexual abuse and adult psychiatric illness.[51] The meta-analysis includes 17 studies and finds that those with a history of maltreatment in these longitudinal studies were significantly more likely to develop anxiety, depression, eating disorders, PTSD, and reported suicide attempts. Included in the analysis is the Christchurch Health and Development Study from New Zealand, a birth cohort of more than 1200 individuals. By age 25 years, those with a history of childhood sexual abuse were 2.4 times more likely to suffer from mental health problems, even after controlling for other known variables that increase one's risk for the development of mental illness.[52] Similar findings on the long-term mental health effects among victims of childhood maltreatment are reported in multiple large-scale studies (see **Table 1**).

Children who have experienced one childhood adversity or have experienced a given abuse are significantly more likely than other children to experience multiple adversities and abuses.[53,54] Furthermore, as can be noted from the previous discussion, there is significant overlap in the symptoms and sequelae of childhood physical, sexual, and psychological maltreatment. Recently, population-based studies addressing mental health outcomes have examined the effect of multiple forms of childhood abuse and adversity. Green and colleagues[54] analyzed data from the National Comorbidity Survey, a nationally representative sample of adults, to look at the correlations between childhood adversity and the development of mental illness in childhood and adulthood. The study included approximately 5700 individuals who were evaluated for 12 different adversities including physical and sexual abuse. In general, the data suggest that childhood adversities are associated with nearly half of all childhood-onset psychiatric disorders, and between one-fourth and one-third of all later-onset disorders. In multivariate analysis, childhood physical and sexual abuse were independently associated with statistically significant increases in rates of mood, anxiety, substance use, and disruptive behavior disorders, accounting for between 50% and 100% increased risk for a specific cluster of psychiatric illnesses (reported odds ratios of 1.5–2.1).

Initially researchers developed a conceptual model to explain the observed association, with the hypothesis that adverse childhood experiences affects child development, resulting in behaviors that increase the likelihood of developing risk factors for common physical and mental diseases.[39] However, subsequent analyses of the data demonstrates that for many of the conditions, such as lung cancer, chronic obstructive pulmonary disease, and liver disease, even when one controls for behavioral risk factors there is still an increase in the rates of disease among those with multiple childhood adversities.[55–57]

Research demonstrating health problems in children with a history of childhood maltreatment provides additional evidence that increased rates of illness do not solely result from developing risky behaviors. Flaherty and colleagues[58,59] analyzed data from the Consortium for Longitudinal Studies of Child Abuse and Neglect (LONG-SCAN), a data set that includes more than 1300 at-risk children recruited from 5 centers throughout the United States. Their analysis focused on the effects of adverse childhood exposure on health at 6 and then at 12 years of age. The participants in the LONGSCAN study (parent/child dyads) were interviewed at 4, 6, 8, and 12 years of age, and the population was heavily weighted toward individuals who were more likely to experience adversity. By the time the children were 6 years old, 67% had experienced at least one adverse event.[58] Among 6-year-olds, having one adverse exposure doubled the risk for overall poor health, and 4 or more adverse exposures tripled the likelihood of illness compared with children without reported adversities. By the second phase of the study at age 12, only 10% had no adverse childhood event, and more than 20% experienced 5 or more types of childhood adversity.[59] Participants who had 5 or more adverse childhood events were at significantly increased risk of having any health complaint. In children 6 to 12 years old, increased somatic complaints, overall poor health as reported by the child and illnesses requiring a doctor's visit, correlated with increased adverse experiences.[59] The investigators' interpretation was that an increased number of adversities (allostatic load) as well as time (older children had more health problems) contributed to the correlations observed in their data analysis.[59]

These large, population-based studies and meta-analyses provide important new evidence that medical and mental health complications are more frequently observed in children and adults who have a history of childhood maltreatment. Several biological models have been proposed that may explain some of the observed findings between childhood adversity and long-term health outcomes. Most of these studies look for neuroendocrine changes that are part of or regulated by aspects of the hypothalamic-pituitary-adrenal (HPA) axis.[60,61] Although specific findings between studies vary, in general there is good evidence that exposure to childhood maltreatment correlates with long-lasting dysregulation of the HPA axis.[62,63] Such findings among abused individuals add further evidence that long-term medical and psychological outcomes are not merely a function of maladaptive behaviors but also result from physiologic changes caused by childhood maltreatment.

FORENSIC EVALUATION

The forensic evaluation of a maltreated child is an essential component for estimating the damage to that child. The American Academy of Child and Adolescent Psychiatry (AACAP) published *Practice Parameters for the Forensic Evaluation of Child and*

Adolescents Who May Have Been Physically or Sexually Abused in 1997.[64] These parameters were developed through an extensive literature review and consensus process. The parameters refer to the earlier AACAP *Guidelines for the Clinical Evaluation of Child and Adolescent Sexual Abuse*[65] and the *Guidelines for the Psychosocial Evaluation of Suspected Sexual Abuse in Young Children* developed by the American Professional Society on the Abuse of Children (APSAC),[66] along with two additional APSAC guidelines addressing the use of anatomic dolls[67] and evaluating suspected psychological maltreatment.[68] APSAC published revised guidelines on the *Psychosocial Evaluation of Suspected Sexual Abuse in Children* in 1997.[69] At present, AACAP is finalizing a Practice Parameter on Forensic Evaluations that will likely appear in 2011.

These AACAP Practice Parameters and APSAC Guidelines provide useful information and perspectives for improving the quality of forensic evaluations seeking to estimate damage to victims of child maltreatment. As described in these practice guidelines, thorough forensic evaluation consists of reviewing all relevant investigative, medical, mental health, school, and legal records, interviewing the child and child's caregivers, and often others with first-hand observations and knowledge of the child.

Many experts believe that the electronic recording of forensic interviews of children who may have been sexually abused should be a standard of practice. The first author of this article (D.L.C.), who has 30 years of experience of recording interviews with sexually abused children on video, has found these recorded interviews very useful in assuring the accuracy of the information he relies on for writing reports and illustrating the basis for his testimony in trials. Electronic recording protects subjects in these evaluations from errors in citing their statements and behaviors, and protects the evaluator from allegations of misrepresentation. In cases involving multiple victims, transcription at the time of the interview has also proved useful in preparing for depositions and trial testimony. These cases often contain large amounts of information and can proceed slowly over months or years. Having both recordings and transcripts available during preparation for testimony is very useful.

In addition to these sources of information, there are several psychological instruments that were specifically developed for use with traumatized and maltreated children. Among these are the Child Sexual Behavior Inventory,[70] Social Behavior Inventory,[71] the Expectations Test,[72] Trauma Symptom Checklist—Children,[73] and the Trauma Symptom Checklist for Young Children.[74] The inclusion of these psychological tests in a forensic evaluation provides a standardized way to compare the child with other children of similar age and gender with and without histories of maltreatment. A few of these also include validity scales, which can be useful for assessing overreporting and underreporting of symptoms and behaviors. Although these tests are useful for assessing a child's present symptoms, functioning, and present treatment needs, they do not predict future medical or mental health sequelae.

There is great value in collaboration with psychologists and other professionals who can assist in reviewing records, participating in interviews, conducting psychological testing, and interpreting medical findings. A team approach provides an opportunity for discussing the complexity of these evaluations, controls for bias, and opens the process to professional training.

A child's initial reaction to experiences of maltreatment may be the best evidence available to a forensic evaluator to determine present impact and to estimate the risk for ongoing difficulties. However, some children may be resilient to a specific abusive experience, and a "sleeper" or "psychological time bomb" effect has been noted among a significant number of longitudinally studied victims of child maltreatment. In such situations there are few or no discernible initial reactions of the kind often found in maltreated children, but significant problems develop later in the individual's life that may be related to the earlier maltreatment.

RECOMMENDATIONS FOR PRESENT AND FUTURE TREATMENT

Bernet and Corwin[75] collaborated on an article describing the application of scientific evidence regarding the long-term harms of child sexual abuse to the forensic questions raised in a civil lawsuit involving the sexual abuse of a teenage boy by his school counselor. Present and future treatment recommendations along with their levels of certainty are discussed in that article.

There are now well-established evidence-based treatments for sexually and physically abused children. Trauma-focused cognitive-behavior therapy (TF-CBT)[76] and alternatives for families: a cognitive-behavioral therapy (AF-CBT)[32] are 2 examples with strong evidence of effectiveness and well-written training manuals, books, and other training resources.[77] Recommendations for evidence-based therapy, support for caregivers, and approaches that address learning and social problems are among interventions that forensic mental health experts should consider. Opportunities for future treatment courses should be considered in light of the growing evidence for long-term harms, as already described. Even though effective treatment reduces symptoms and dysfunction, it does not remove the memory of and all other traces of maltreatment. It will be many years or decades before we know how effective these and future treatments are in preventing and reducing the long-term harms associated with child maltreatment and other childhood adversities.

ESTIMATING OVERALL LIFETIME DAMAGE

Estimating the total cost of lifetime care to ameliorate the known harms of child maltreatment and to compensate victims for the other losses and suffering associated with being maltreated is beyond the expertise of child psychiatrists or other mental health professionals alone. Vocational experts and health economists contribute their perspectives and expertise in translating the known harms associated with child maltreatment, considering the increased risk for future psychiatric and medical problems and, in some cases, diminished educational achievement and lowered earning capacity. Ultimately, it is beyond the expertise of any professional expert to determine the noneconomic losses including pain, suffering, diminished joy and satisfaction in life, interpersonal problems, and years of life lost to medical problems more common among people maltreated during childhood. However, it is incumbent on the forensic expert to explain current behaviors and future medical and mental health risks borne by victims of child maltreatment in a scientifically rigorous manner, so that judges and juries can make well-informed decisions regarding damage and associated costs. Child maltreatment places a burden on victims, making them more susceptible to subsequent stressors in life. Ultimately, in those cases that do not resolve before trials, juries will weigh the admissible evidence, and consider the credibility of both fact and expert witnesses before deciding what is just.

ACKNOWLEDGMENTS

The authors wish to acknowledge the assistance of Professor John E.B. Myers, editor of The APSAC Handbook on Child Maltreatment, Third Edition (2011), for providing an early copy of that publication for use and reference in preparing this article. Assistance by the Primary Children's Medical Center library in performing literature searches and obtaining articles cited in this publication was invaluable.

REFERENCES

1. Kempe CH, Silverman FN, Steele BF, et al. The battered child syndrome. JAMA 1962;181:17–24.
2. Summit RC. The child sexual abuse accommodation syndrome. Child Abuse Negl 1983;7(2):177–93.
3. Olafson E, Corwin DL, Summit RC. Modern history of child sexual abuse awareness: cycles of discovery and suppression. Child Abuse Negl 1993;17(1):7–24.
4. Bohn DK, Holz KA. Sequelae of abuse. Health effects of childhood sexual abuse, domestic battering, and rape. J Nurse Midwifery 1996;41(6):442–56.
5. King WJ, MacKay M, Sirnick A, et al. Shaken baby syndrome in Canada: clinical characteristics and outcomes of hospital cases. Can Med Assoc J 2003;168(2):155–9.
6. Silver JM, Kramer R, Greenwald S, et al. The association between head injuries and psychiatric disorders: findings from the New Haven NIMH Epidemiologic Catchment Area Study. Brain Inj 2001;15(11):935–45.
7. The economic cost of spinal cord injury and traumatic brain injury in Australia. Geelong (Australia): Access Economics for The Victorian Neurotrauma Initiative; June 2009.
8. Johnson CF. Child sexual abuse. Lancet 2004;364(9432):462–70.
9. Felitti VJ. Childhood sexual abuse, depression, and family dysfunction in adult obese patients: a case control study. South Med J 1993;86(7):732–6.
10. Heitkemper M, Jarrett M, Taylor P, et al. Effect of sexual and physical abuse on symptom experiences in women with irritable bowel syndrome. Nurs Res 2001;50(1):15–23.
11. Carpenter MT, Hugler R, Enzenauer RJ, et al. Physical and sexual abuse in female patients with fibromyalgia. J Clin Rheumatol 1998;4(6):301–6.
12. Latthe P, Mignini L, Gray R, et al. Factors predisposing women to chronic pelvic pain: systematic review. BMJ 2006;332(7544):749–55.
13. Chartier MJ, Walker JR, Naimark B. Childhood abuse, adult health, and health care utilization: results from a representative community sample. Am J Epidemiol 2007;165(9):1031–8.
14. Berliner L. Child sexual abuse: definitions, prevalence and consequences. In: Myers JE, editor. The APSAC handbook on child maltreatment. 3rd edition. Thousand Oaks (CA): Sage; 2011. p. 215–32.
15. McLeer SV, Deblinger E, Henry D, et al. Sexually abused children at high risk for posttraumatic stress disorder. J Am Acad Child Adolesc Psychiatry 1992;31:875–9.
16. Dubner AE, Motta RW. Sexually and physically abused foster care children and posttraumatic stress disorder. J Consult Clin Psychol 1999;67:367–73.
17. Deblinger E, McLeer SV, Atkins MS, et al. Post-traumatic stress in sexually abused, physically abused, and non-abused children. Child Abuse Negl 1989;13:403–8.
18. Kendall-Tackett KA, Williams LM, Finkelhor D. Impact of sexual abuse on children: a review and synthesis of recent empirical studies. Psychol Bull 1993;113(1):164–80.
19. Spartaro J, Mullen PE, Burgess PM, et al. Impact of child sexual abuse on mental health: prospective study in males and females. Br J Psychiatry 2004;184:416–21.
20. Brown J, Cohen JA, Johnson JG, et al. Childhood abuse and neglect: specificity of effects on adolescent on adolescents and young adult depression and suicidality. J Am Acad Child Adolesc Psychiatry 1999;38:1490–6.

21. Spatz-Widom C, Brzustowicz LM. MAOA and the "cycle of violence": childhood abuse and neglect, MAOA genotype, and risk for violent and anti-social behavior. Biol Psychiatry 2006;60:684–9.
22. Feiring C, Taska L, Lewis M. Age and gender differences in children's and adolescents' adaptation to sexual abuse. Child Abuse Negl 1999;23(2):115–28.
23. Cohen JA, Mannarino AP. A treatment study for sexually abused preschool children: outcome during a one-year follow-up. J Am Acad Child Adolesc Psychiatry 1997;36(9):1228–35.
24. Brilleslijper-Kater SN, Friedrich WN, Corwin DL. Sexual knowledge and emotional reactions as indicators of sexual abuse in young children: theory and research challenges. Child Abuse Negl 2004;28(10):1007–17.
25. Cohen JA, Perel LM, DeBellis MD, et al. Treating traumatized children: clinical implications of the psychobiology of posttraumatic stress disorder. Trauma Violence Abuse 2002;3:91–108.
26. Teicher MH, Andersen SL, Polcari A, et al. Developmental neurobiology of childhood stress and trauma. Psychiatr Clin North Am 2002;25(2):397–426, vii–viii.
27. Weber DA, Reynolds CR. Clinical perspectives on neurobiological effects of psychological trauma. Neuropsychol Rev 2004;14(2):115–29.
28. Endo T, Sugiyama T, Someya T. Attention-deficit/hyperactivity disorder and dissociative disorder among abused children. Psychiatry Clin Neurosci 2006;60(4):434–8.
29. Runyon MK, Urquiza AJ. Child physical abuse: interventions for parents who engage in coercive parenting practices and their children. In: Myers JE, editor. The APSAC handbook on child maltreatment. 3rd edition. Thousand Oaks (CA): Sage; 2011. p. 193–212.
30. Saunders BE, Berliner L, Hanson RF. Child physical and sexual abuse: guidelines for treatment (final report: January 15, 2004). Charleston (SC): National Crime Victims Research and Treatment Center; 2004.
31. Runyon MK, Deblinger E, Schroeder CM. Pilot evaluation of outcomes of combined parent-child cognitive-behavioral group therapy for families at risk for child physical abuse. Cognit Behav Pract 2009;16:101–18.
32. Kolko DJ, Swenson CC. Assessing and treating physically abused children and their families: a cognitive behavioral approach. Thousand Oaks (CA): Sage; 2002.
33. Hart SN, Brassard MR, Davidson HA, et al. Psychological maltreatment. In: Myers JE, editor. Child maltreatment. 3rd edition. Los Angeles (CA), London, New Delhi, Singapore, Washington, DC: Sage; 2011. p. 125–44.
34. Hart SN, Brassard MR. Definition of psychological maltreatment. Indianapolis: Office for the Study of the Psychological Rights of the Child. Bloomington (IN): Indiana University School of Education; 1991, 2001.
35. Hart SN, Binggeli NJ, Brassard MR. Evidence of the effects of psychological maltreatment. J Emot Abuse 1998;1(1):27–58.
36. Binggeli NJ, Hart SN, Brassard MR. Psychological maltreatment: a study guide. Thousand Oaks (CA): Sage; 2000.
37. Brassard MM, Donovan KL. Defining psychological maltreatment. In: Feerick MM, Knutson JF, Trickett PK, et al, editors. Child abuse and neglect: definitions, classification, and a framework for research. Baltimore (MD): Paul H. Brookes; 2006. p. 151–97.
38. Krugman RD, Krugman MK. Emotional abuse in the classroom. The pediatrician's role in diagnosis and treatment. Am J Dis Child 1984;138(3):284–6.

39. Felitti VJ, Anda RF, Nordenberg D, et al. Relationship of childhood abuse and household dysfunction to many of the leading causes of death in adults. The Adverse Childhood Experiences (ACE) Study. Am J Prev Med 1998;14(4):245–58.
40. Wegman HL, Stetler C. A meta-analytic review of the effects of childhood abuse on medical outcomes in adulthood. Psychosom Med 2009;71(8):805–12.
41. Cohen J. Statistical power analysis for the behavioral sciences. 2nd edition. Hillsdale (NJ): Lawrence Erlbaum Associates; 1988.
42. Dube SR, Cook ML, Edwards VJ. Health-related outcomes of adverse childhood experiences in Texas, 2002. Prev Chronic Dis 2010;7(3):A52.
43. Springer KW, Sheridan J, Kuo D, et al. Long-term physical and mental health consequences of childhood physical abuse: results from a large population-based sample of men and women. Child Abuse Negl 2007;31(5):517–30.
44. Irish L, Kobayashi I, Delahanty DL. Long-term physical health consequences of childhood sexual abuse: a meta-analytic review. J Pediatr Psychol 2010;35(5): 450–61.
45. Yehuda R, Halligan SL, Grossman R. Childhood trauma and risk for PTSD: relationship to intergenerational effects of trauma, parental PTSD, and cortisol excretion. Dev Psychopathol 2001;13(3):733–53.
46. Mancini C, Van Ameringen M, MacMillan H. Relationship of childhood sexual and physical abuse to anxiety disorders. J Nerv Ment Dis 1995;183(5):309–14.
47. Gladstone G, Parker G, Wilhelm K, et al. Characteristics of depressed patients who report childhood sexual abuse. Am J Psychiatry 1999;156(3):431–7.
48. Brown GR, McBride L, Bauer MS, et al. Impact of childhood abuse on the course of bipolar disorder: a replication study in U.S. veterans. J Affect Disord 2005; 89(1–3):57–67.
49. Read J, van Os J, Morrison AP, et al. Childhood trauma, psychosis and schizophrenia: a literature review with theoretical and clinical implications. Acta Psychiatr Scand 2005;112(5):330–50.
50. Molnar BE, Buka SL, Kessler RC. Child sexual abuse and subsequent psychopathology: results from the National Comorbidity Survey. Am J Public Health 2001; 91(5):753–60.
51. Chen LP, Murad MH, Paras ML, et al. Sexual abuse and lifetime diagnosis of psychiatric disorders: systematic review and meta-analysis. Mayo Clin Proc 2010;85(7):618–29.
52. Fergusson DM, Boden JM, Horwood LJ. Exposure to childhood sexual and physical abuse and adjustment in early adulthood. Child Abuse Negl 2008;32(6): 607–19.
53. Dong M, Anda RF, Felitti VJ, et al. The interrelatedness of multiple forms of childhood abuse, neglect, and household dysfunction. Child Abuse Negl 2004;28(7): 771–84.
54. Green JG, McLaughlin KA, Berglund PA, et al. Childhood adversities and adult psychiatric disorders in the national comorbidity survey replication I: associations with first onset of DSM-IV disorders. Arch Gen Psychiatry 2010;67(2):113–23.
55. Dong M, Dube SR, Felitti VJ, et al. Adverse childhood experiences and self-reported liver disease: new insights into the causal pathway. Arch Intern Med 2003;163(16):1949–56.
56. Anda RF, Brown DW, Dube SR, et al. Adverse childhood experiences and chronic obstructive pulmonary disease in adults. Am J Prev Med 2008;34(5):396–403.
57. Brown DW, Anda RF, Felitti VJ, et al. Adverse childhood experiences are associated with the risk of lung cancer: a prospective cohort study. BMC Public Health 2010;10:20.

58. Flaherty EG, Thompson R, Litrownik AJ, et al. Effect of early childhood adversity on child health. Arch Pediatr Adolesc Med 2006;160(12):1232–8.

59. Flaherty EG, Thompson R, Litrownik AJ, et al. Adverse childhood exposures and reported child health at age 12. Acad Pediatr 2009;9(3):150–6.

60. De Bellis MD. Developmental traumatology: the psychobiological development of maltreated children and its implications for research, treatment, and policy. Dev Psychopathol 2001;13(3):539–64.

61. Neigh GN, Gillespie CF, Nemeroff CB. The neurobiological toll of child abuse and neglect. Trauma Violence Abuse 2009;10(4):389–410.

62. Trickett PK, Noll JG, Susman EJ, et al. Attenuation of cortisol across development for victims of sexual abuse. Dev Psychopathol 2010;22(1):165–75.

63. Carpenter LL, Carvalho JP, Tyrka AR, et al. Decreased adrenocorticotropic hormone and cortisol responses to stress in healthy adults reporting significant childhood maltreatment. Biol Psychiatry 2007;62(10):1080–7.

64. American Academy of Child & Adolescent Psychiatry. Practice parameters for the forensic evaluation of children and adolescents who may have been physically or sexually abused. J Am Acad Child Adolesc Psychiatry 1997;36:423–42.

65. American Academy of Child & Adolescent Psychiatry. Guidelines for the clinical evaluation of child and adolescent sexual abuse. J Am Acad Child Adolesc Psychiatry 1988;27:655–7.

66. American Professional Society on the Abuse of Children. Psychosocial evaluation of suspected sexual abuse in young children. Chicago (IL): American Professional Society on the Abuse of Children; 1990.

67. American Professional Society on the Abuse of Children. Guidelines for the use of anatomical dolls in child sexual abuse assessments. Chicago (IL): American Professional Society on the Abuse of Children; 1995.

68. American Professional Society on the Abuse of Children. Guidelines for the psychosocial evaluation of suspected psychological maltreatment. Chicago (IL): American Professional Society on the Abuse of Children; 1995.

69. American Professional Society on the Abuse of Children. Psychosocial evaluation of suspected sexual abuse in children. 2nd edition. Chicago (IL): American Professional Society on the Abuse of Children; 1997.

70. Friedrich WN. Child sexual behavior inventory. Lutz (FL): Psychological Assessment Resources; 1997.

71. Gully KJ. Social behavior inventory: professional manual. Salt Lake City (UT): PEAK Ascent; 2003.

72. Gully KJ. Expectation test: professional manual. Salt Lake City (UT): PEAK Ascent; 2003.

73. Briere J. Trauma symptom checklist—children. Lutz (FL): Psychological Assessment Resources; 1996.

74. Briere J. Trauma symptom checklist for children. Lutz (FL): Psychological Assessment Resources; 2005.

75. Bernet W, Corwin D. An evidence-based approach for estimating present and future damages from child sexual abuse. J Am Acad Psychiatry Law 2006; 34(2):224–30.

76. Cohen JA, Mannarino AP, Deblinger E. Treating trauma and traumatic grief in children and adolescents. New York: The Guilford Press; 2006.

77. National Child Traumatic Stress Network. Available at: www.nctsn.net. Accessed October 1, 2010.

Forensic Psychiatry in France: The Outreau Case and False Allegations of Child Sexual Abuse

Paul Bensussan, MD*,1

KEYWORDS

- Outreau • Child sexual abuse • False allegations
- Psychiatric expertise • Psychological expertise

Outreau is a small town in the north of France. The Outreau case entered the media in May 2001 in a commonplace manner: a sordid story of incest in an underprivileged social class. However, numerous revelations would change the nature of this case until the trial in May 2004. The allegations became more serious and the number of victims increased. The findings of the psychiatric and psychological experts who examined the children before the trial left no doubt: the children were not liars. That was also the view of the *juge d'instruction*, the investigating judge.

This article examines the joint mechanisms that created a state of confusion in the roles of the judge and the experts. In the words of Hubert van Gijseghem, this resulted in the expert "sitting in the chair of the judge."[1] In this case, the psychiatric expertise constituted most of the evidence that favored the prosecution. The prosecution experts validated the narratives of the children and attributed "traits of a pedophiliac or pervert" to each of the accused. The author of this article was honored to be summoned as a witness for the defendants to provide the *Cour d'assises* the French criminal court, with a critical examination of the expert opinions submitted against the accused.

This article starts with a purely factual summary of this historical case. Then, the author's analysis illustrates, in numerous respects, the failings of child protection and its catastrophic influence on the operation of the judicial system.[2] The author further challenges militant dogma and erroneous beliefs that have resulted in child protection, at least in France, constituting a true sexual exception in the law, that is,

The author has nothing to disclose.
Private practice, Versailles, France
1 National Psychiatric Expert appointed by the *Cour de cassation* (the French Supreme Court).
* 13 rue de la Pourvoirie, 78000 Versailles, France.
E-mail address: mail@paulbensussan.fr

Child Adolesc Psychiatric Clin N Am 20 (2011) 519–532
doi:10.1016/j.chc.2011.03.002
1056-4993/11/$ – see front matter © 2011 Elsevier Inc. All rights reserved.

childpsych.theclinics.com

an area in which the fundamental principles of criminal law (presumption of innocence, burden of proof on the prosecution) are not applied or are inoperative. The author offers some lessons to be learned from the Outreau case in light of comparisons with the Anglo-Saxon judicial system. To improve the handling of word-against-word cases, in which evidence is often lacking, there must be joint collaboration between judges and experts. In the words of a member of the French Parliament speaking before the Parliamentary Board of Inquiry that was ordered, after the trial, to examine the causes of dysfunction in the Outreau case, "The tragedy is that the procedure was complied with. If this were not so, it would be so simple."[3]

SUMMARY OF THE OUTREAU CASE

This summary is based on evidence submitted at trial and a book, La Méprise [The Error], by a French journalist, Florence Aubenas.[4]

The Disclosure

The initial disclosure occurred in September 2000. At first, it was a simple story that started with the revelation, at school, of incest committed by parents on their 4 sons, who were between 4 and 10 years of age. The alleged rapes were revealed at the start of the new school year by the exhibitionistic behavior of the oldest son during class, who put a pencil in his behind. The initial story was frightening: ogres and ogresses who abused little children for years, subjecting them to zoophilic rape. According to the early accounts, several children had been murdered and buried during these parties. An avalanche of revelations ensued. The 4 children who had been placed in foster families and subjected to the most suggestive questions revealed an impressive list of alleged abusers and child victims.

On the day after her arrest, the mother of the children, Myriam Badaoui, confessed to the incestuous rapes committed by her husband, Thierry Delay, acknowledging her complicity. As legal proceedings commenced on December 5, 2000, the young juge d'instruction (investigative judge) Fabrice Burgaud, took this case very seriously. (In France, the legal system is inquisitorial rather than adversarial. That is, the juge d'instruction is in charge of conducting the investigation, preparing the case, and assessing whether it should proceed to trial.) France had been affected by the Dutroux case, named after the pedophilic predator who raped, confined, and assassinated several young girls in Belgium during the 1990s. In the Outreau case, Judge Burgaud was determined and convinced that "the children were not liars." He would repeat this phrase hundreds of times until the end of the investigative phase of the proceedings. The truth would be revealed at a later time.

The Escalation

The case escalated at dawn on March 6, 2001. In a spectacular crackdown, similar to a drug or antiterrorism raid, approximately 60 neighbors of the Delay-Badaoui family were questioned, taken to the police station, and placed in custody. Alleged victims and alleged abusers found themselves together in the early hours of the morning.

At that stage of the investigation, 16 children were questioned by policemen untrained in interviewing children. They were asked questions such as, "Did men or women do nasty things to you?" and, "Have you ever seen your daddy's weenie?" The children were asked to point out the adults who had abused them from among the portraits shown to them. No methodological precautions were taken. Because all the photographs were of adult suspects, each adult pointed out became a guilty party.

The foster mothers of the 4 brothers often phoned each other to compare new revelations from their respective protégés. That led to other adults being subsequently placed in temporary detention: the baker; the Abbé Dominique Wiel; the bailiff and his wife; and the taxi driver, Martel, who drove the children to the farm in Belgium where they were allegedly raped by all kinds of animals. The Belgian lead and that of the respectable abusers of poor children were then pursued.

Myriam Badaoui, who was confident in the promise made by her lawyer as to her imminent release, decided to collaborate with the judge. Her imagination showed no bounds: "The children gave names. The judge would come to fetch me [in the remand center] and would tell me that it was true. I believed him and so continued to follow him. I thought it unfair for me to carry the burden alone." No one dared to point out the contradictions or incoherencies in Ms Badaoui's statements. The lawyers failed to suspect any mythomaniac tendencies, nor were they diagnosed by the experts. (Mythomania refers to habitual or compulsive lying, which is also called pathologic lying and pseudologia fantastica.) Ms Badaoui then wrote 10 or so letters to the investigative judge in which she expressed her surprise at remaining in temporary detention: Had she spoken in vain?

In July 2001, a new order provided for the temporary placement of 25 additional children. "Most of these children seemed traumatized" recalled one of the police officers. "But we asked ourselves why: Was it from having suffered sexual molestation or having been brutally ripped away from their families?" The case grew every day. Confrontations, in which alleged victims and alleged abusers were questioned face to face in front of the judge to explain their differing accounts of the facts, were organized in groups. All requests for individual confrontations submitted by the defense were refused. Those denials were upheld by the *Chambre de l'instruction* (the investigative court), that is, the appellate court responsible for reviewing the decisions of the investigative judge.

The Explosion

On January 10, 2002, the case took an even more spectacular turn. One of the accused, Mr Daniel Legrand, decided to prove his innocence by the most absurd means: "I wanted to tempt the devil and to find something more intelligent to bring out their lies...." Mr Legrand consequently told the investigators that Ms Badaoui's husband, Mr Thierry Delay, not only raped but also killed a small Belgian girl (like in the Dutroux case) and buried her in the allotment gardens. Contrary to all expectations, Ms Badaoui confirmed those imaginary statements. Even better, she further provided the judge with all of the details of that murder. Diggers began excavating the indicated area under the horrified eyes of onlookers and television cameras.

France held its breath. At that point, 10 or so child protection agencies decided to get involved in the case. (Under French law, an agency may be joined as a civil party in proceedings related to its field, which has the perverse effect of attracting agencies to cases that do not directly concern them, notably in matters attracting heavy media attention.) The Minister of the Interior visited the scene. Also, Ms Ségolène Royal, a future candidate in the 2007 presidential election, launched her pedophilia prevention campaign with much hype. The slogan for her campaign was *Se taire, c'est laisser faire* (To say nothing is to do nothing). No murdered child was ever found buried in the gardens of Outreau.

In such an elaborate complex case with a total lack of hard evidence and full of inconsistencies, psychiatric and psychological expertise becomes indispensable. However, the psychiatric and psychological evaluations may confirm, without qualification, the statements of the children and may become evidence condemning the accused. Of the 17 children alleged to be victims, all were deemed to be perfectly credible. With respect to the adults who admitted and reported certain acts, the real issue was whether they had mythomaniac tendencies. However, the psychiatric and psychological experts also deemed these individuals to be perfectly credible and genuine; adults who denied involvement in criminal acts reflected all the traits of sexual abusers, according to the psychiatric and psychological experts.

The Trial: A Legal Shipwreck

The trial, which began in May 2004, was a legal shipwreck. By that time, almost all of the accused had been in temporary detention between 2 and 3 years. The media coverage was enormous. Seventeen adults were in the accused box: 3 made accusations, 1 said nothing at all, and 13 denied all allegations. Having come to see monsters, journalists were swayed during the proceedings by accused individuals who cried more than the victims, combined with numerous about turns, retractions, and inconsistencies. The press and public opinion soon asked for clemency with the same vigor they had previously called for lynching.

At the trial, Ms Marie-Christine Gryson-Dejehansart, the psychological expert who examined 16 of the children and head of a child protection agency, proved to be incompetent and was unable to respond to questions posed by Maître Dupond-Moretti, counsel for the defense. She was jeered as she left the courtroom.

However, as the trial continued, an extraordinary development occurred. Ms Myriam Badaoui, the principal accuser, retracted all of her allegations. Before a dumbfounded courtroom, Ms Badaoui admitted to having lied from the moment of her arrest. She asked to be pardoned, one by one, by each person she had accused, regretting that she had destroyed their lives. She said, "Nothing is true! I am a sick person and a liar!"

When the presiding judge asked Ms Badaoui whether the children lied, she responded, "They don't lie, but sometimes they make mistakes!" However, the investigative judge, Fabrice Burgaud, did not express any doubt or any regret about primarily relying on the word of a mythomaniac and her children during the course of his investigation. He stated feebly, "It is not true that everything was invented. The only thing is that verifications were conducted in vain."

The absurdity of the case and of the investigation was clear. Among the 13 adults claiming their innocence, the general public prosecutor asked that 7 be acquitted and the other 6 be convicted. Nothing was said relating to 1 of the accused, who committed suicide in his cell after writing an emotional letter to Judge Burgaud in which he claimed his innocence. The jury rendered a verdict in accordance with directions of the *Parquet* (the public prosecutor), a verdict described as unreadable and incomprehensible by the press, giving the impression of a true drawing of lots of the accused.

The convictions in the Outreau case were appealed to the *Cour de cassation* (Criminal Court) and the trial opened in Paris in November 2005. On November 17, 2005, the expert Jean-Luc Viaux was strongly attacked by counsel for the defense and also by the general public prosecutor; a rare occurrence. Mr Viaux left the hearing furious and greatly frustrated to face a forest of microphones and cameras. He chose that moment on leaving the hearing to question the mediocre remuneration for criminal expert reports in France. Mr Viaux's historic remark—"When one pays experts at the same rate as a cleaning lady, one receives expert reports of a cleaning lady"—greatly irritated the Minister of Justice, who requested at the end of the trial that Mr Viaux be removed from the list of experts. However, if the fees of French experts do not constitute an attenuating circumstance, it is relevant to inform our American colleagues of the specific remuneration provided for such important expert assessments: 170 euros per child, which includes the hearings, the preparation of the report, and all filings in the criminal court. This work is a true calling.

On November 18, 2005, the author of this article testified at the *Cour d'assises* as a witness for the defense. The author conducted a methodological examination of the expert reports prepared by his colleagues and noted the failures and overzealousness that, in his opinion, resulted in the case taking on such proportions. According to the newspaper, *Le Monde,* he "dealt the final blow."[5] The author specifically pointed out that convicting adults without any evidence other than the word of the children is, in the end, tantamount to giving the children life sentences. That is, the justice system irreversibly conferred on them the status of victims.[6]

The 6 individuals who had been convicted at first instance were acquitted on December 1, 2005, by the *Cour d'assises* of Paris. France was in a daze. Beyond the judicial error of the court of first instance, the faith of each citizen in justice had been shattered. In the weeks following the announcement of the verdict, the Minister of Justice, conscious of the scope of this case extending beyond simply that of a judicial error, ordered the establishment of a "Parliamentary Commission of Inquiry to investigate the dysfunction of justice in the Outreau case." Two substantive questions were addressed to all members of the Commission: What really happened during the Outreau case? How could other Outreau-type cases be avoided in the future?

WHY DID THE OUTREAU SHIPWRECK OCCUR?

Probably all criminal lawyers have acted in Outreau-type cases in the past and will continue to do so in the future. It is common for defendants to be convicted in word-against-word cases without hard evidence, even if it leaves lawyers bitter and outraged at the subjectivity of psychiatric expertise condemning their clients or sanctifying the word of the child. How do we understand that we needed the Outreau case was needed to shake certainties? Few people in France had warned against the risk that an easily influenced judicial machine might get carried away. By what incredible hypocrisy did we pretend to discover in 2004 that the word of a child could be fragile, especially if the child was very young, had experienced atrocities, and furthermore had been poorly interrogated? What conditions enabled such an obvious fact to finally surface?

Did the examination of the facts contradict the statements of the victims? Did a judicial confrontation identify signs of insincerity in the accusing adults or in the children? Were the accused in a position to prove their innocence? Did the experts reveal flaws or incoherencies or criticize the manner in which information was obtained? Not at all. In any case, a retraction by a child does not attract the same interest as the first revelation. The explanation given for a retraction simply denotes the weight of guilt or a common ambivalence with respect to the alleged abuser. Rarely does a judge request an expert opinion on the reliability of a retraction.[7]

Two conditions were key in establishing awareness of the fallibility of children's statements and experts' opinions and creating a state of shock. First, the retraction did not come from a child. At the hearing on May 18, 2004, it was Ms Myriam Badaoui, mother of the child victims and principal accuser, who exculpated those whom she had implicated in the case. Her turnaround was ephemeral: she went back on this retraction at the following hearing, changing her story once again. That led not only the lawyers and judges in the case but also journalists and public opinion to realize the extent of her mythomania and of the damage caused.

Second, the retraction did not call into question the victim status of the children, at least for a certain number of them. Despite many adults being wrongly accused, the

4 children of the Delay-Badaoui couple were still serious victims of incestuous rape. Only the other children became imaginary victims.

Without these 2 conditions (the second, in particular), the Outreau case would have had a lesser impact or none at all. No commission of inquiry would have been created to examine the dysfunction of justice and most of the accused would be serving harsh sentences. It was that sudden new development that led public opinion, the judges, and the media to recognize the fragile nature of the word of children, not to mention that of experts.

Comments by Government

It was previously known that psychiatric and psychological expertise was fallible, but the Outreau judges pretended to ignore that fact, giving experts and their science excessive credit. For example, the French Parliament debated the law related to the protection of minors and victims of sexual offenses in June 1998. During that debate, Renaud Dutreil, a Member of Parliament, expressed his concerns: "We are not in a scientific field and the expertise we are speaking of is based largely on interpretation and subjectivity...."

More recently, François Fillon, the current prime minister, posed the following question: "In what other field is it accepted that the accused alone be required to provide evidence of his innocence? No such field exists!" It is clear that, faced with overwhelming evidence provided by mental health experts, an accused is left with only 1 option: proving his or her innocence. That is what lawyers specifically call a reversal of the burden of proof. In principle, this is unacceptable. Under French criminal law, the burden of proof rests on the prosecution. However, in cases of alleged sexual maltreatment of minors in France, a kind of sexual exception applies. That is, evidence that child maltreatment occurred is not required. The alleged victim is deemed to have told the truth. Child advocates say: Can a child be expected to prove the validity of his or her statements?

Dominique Coujard, president of the Criminal Court of Paris, made this lucid but cynical remark: "Judges are just about as confident in experts as experts are in the justice system." Mr Coujard was speaking at a conference organized by an association of fathers, SOS Papa.

Enough of this hypocrisy! Judges knew to what extent psychiatric experts could err, even if they claimed to have only discovered this during the Outreau case. However, it was convenient for them to validate the word of the children by means of psychiatric or psychological expertise. That was what a French psychoanalyst and sociologist called umbrella expertise, which provides greater protection to the person reporting than the minor in danger.[8] Be it the word of children or experts, the Outreau case showed that both were fallible, easily influenced, and abusively established as evidence in a field in which evidence is greatly lacking. As a result of the Outreau case, awareness had been raised and it was alleged that everything would be done to avoid any recurrence of this type of situation; we would see that these good resolutions were not all followed up on.

The Role of Judges

After the Outreau case, both the judge and the experts were criticized. The judge was inexperienced and acted as a psychologically rigid inquisitor, unable to doubt or be open to self-criticism. As a result of this case, the entrance examination for the École Nationale de Magistrature (the National Magistrates' School) has since been altered to include psychological tests and case situations for future judges, to test their ability to question their own certainties.

In France, the investigative judge is a person that Balzac deemed to be the "most powerful man in France."[9] The situation has not evolved significantly since the nineteenth century and the independence of the investigative judge remains complete: no person may give him orders and he is free to conduct any inquiries he deems necessary. More specifically, only the investigative judge can request or refuse a psychiatric or psychological expert, as in the Outreau case. This independence of the investigative judge has been commonly challenged together with the highly sensitive issue relating to the elimination of the role of the investigative judge, which is a personal priority of the current president of France.

However, the judge was far from being the sole player severely criticized at the end of the Outreau trial. In addition, the experts erred unreasonably as they condemned the accused and sanctified the word of the children, which was essentially based on their personal convictions. It is therefore evident that the French courts do not attribute the same importance as the Anglo-Saxon courts to scientific methodology. At the Outreau trial, the list of experts included both scientific psychologists and Lacanian psychoanalysts.

Credibility of Children

Another factor at the Outreau trial was resistance to questioning accusations made by children. There was, above all, the need to believe and the difficulty in standing back when confronted with revelations made by children. Before the Outreau case, and after decades of silence regarding child sexual abuse, one could rightfully believe children who were alleged to be victims. One could not doubt the word of the child, and those such as Dr Hubert van Gijseghem in Canada or this author in France, who pleaded for an examination of the reliability of the revelation, were accused of siding with pedophiles. The state of child protection after the Outreau case is disturbing: did the Outreau case not take us 1 step backward with regard to protecting children?

Credibility is a difficult concept. The entire judicial process is based on the statements of children. The problem is to acknowledge the possibility that, in certain circumstances, the child and his entourage may, in good faith or with destructive intent, provide erroneous or falsified testimony. "In almost all cases, we are therefore not talking about a lie of a child but of a progressive process of contamination of his story from suggestive questioning. In such cases, it is evident that the child, often at pre-school age, is the involuntary victim of a kind of brainwashing, also involuntary."[10] What a French psychologist termed the "process of contamination by questioning"[11] was therefore neglected or overshadowed for years by almost all French experts who agreed, without too much fuss, to allow the judges to ask them the fearsome question relating to credibility and, worse still, to answer such question.

After being heard on November 15, 2004, by the Commission chaired by the *Procureur Général* (Public Prosecutor) Jean-Olivier Viout, immediately following the Outreau trial at the court of first instance, the author reiterated his recommendation that the term credibility be eradicated from the legal jargon and from the mission of the expert. The report provided to the Minister of Justice in February 2005 finally recommended its elimination denouncing its "all too frequent semantic distortion for it to be maintained." The spiral of autosuggestion and error is largely influenced by the principle of precaution. Between the risk of a false-positive (falsely believing in abuse which did not occur) and a false-negative result (not believing a child who makes a revelation), the second result represents, for the professional, the most painful, but also the most dangerous, conscience decision, which raises the question of professional courage: an expert who dares to claim that a revelation is not reliable may err in his judgment, which could have serious consequences. However, experts who choose to systematically incur a false-positive risk (ie, use their expertise to support the relevant allegations however improbable they may be) would be known as protectors of children and would never be unmasked. The impunity of the fainthearted expert would consequently almost be guaranteed because it would take an exceptional case like Outreau and the lunacy of a Myriam Badaoui for him to be uncovered.

Allegations by Children

What has not been said about the child's word? There is the need to believe children to offer them the opportunity to overcome the trauma by means of the therapeutic virtues of the trial. There is a remedial utopia and the distortion of the criminal trial leading to an obligation to convict. However, in reality it is not that simple because the child's word is not always a spoken word and, worse still, does not always come from a child. We are therefore confronted here with a slogan; a short, striking phrase or expression intended to send a message or to support an action, rather than a clinical reality.

It is not always a spoken word from which the revelation originates, but occasionally the allegation is based on behavioral symptoms. However, no symptom exists that is specific to sexual abuse. Another problem is that there is no infallible method for distinguishing children who are victims of abuse from children who are sincerely convinced that they have been abused. In both cases, the narrative, drawings, or tests are impregnated by a sexual theme.

Allegations by Adults

The allegations do not always come from a child. In the Outreau case, observers noted the zeal, but also the tactlessness, with which the child protection workers collected, encouraged, and sometimes even provoked revelations by the children. In numerous cases, particularly with respect to allegations of sexual abuse during conflictual parental separations, 1 parent claims to have obtained a secret. The incubation period of the revelation (marked with suspicions, intuition, interpretation, and domestic questioning) sometimes lasts several months before the judicial process begins. The author emphasizes a recommendation that his working committee provided to the Minister of Justice: in the case of suspicion of intrafamilial sexual assault, the entire family should be subject to an expert assessment and not only the child and the alleged abuser. The parent making the revelation or accusation can shed light on the matter for the expert. The problem is that, in France, in false allegations, no one thinks that the child could be the victim of his own parent's imagination.

This family approach does not come naturally to French investigative judges; their attention seems to focus only on the author/victim couple. It should be pointed out that the coffers of the *Trésor public* (French Treasury Department) are empty and that an additional expert assessment, despite being miserably compensated, is only granted parsimoniously. However, whether abuse occurred or not, the family relations have been disrupted. Why not apply forensic understanding to this systemic analysis?

The Role of Experts

When the child speaks, the situation is more complex. In the case of a spontaneous revelation to a third party outside the family, as in the Outreau case, reliability is high and all signals are red. That is not the case where the revelation is solicited in response to suggestive questions posed by an anxious adult. Militants are not troubled by this type of nuance and the prevailing dogma is at least simple: "The child speaks the truth!" chanted Ségolène Royal, launching her pedophilia prevention campaign in 2002.[12]

In such a demagogic climate, the usefulness of expert assessments in which a child has revealed abuse could be questioned. Only recently, one of the agencies joined as a civil party in the Outreau case strongly called for a presumption of credibility in every case in which the victim was a child. That request was presented in a proposed bill in November 2003 by a group of 71 Members of Parliament. One of the fundamental principles of criminal procedure in France, the presumption of innocence, would have been reversed in cases in which the child was the accuser, creating a sexual exception in law.

With respect to the child's word, the author has always preferred to interpret, decipher, and assess the child's reliability rather than believe in the religious sense of this term. To take a child's word seriously does not mean to take it literally as several unscrupulous fanatics or demagogues have suggested. The author has stated and written numerous times that to lie is to knowingly alter the truth. In an expert assessment, to deem that a revelation is not reliable based on criteria confirmed by scientific literature is not tantamount to treating the child as a liar. Very young children can mix up the real and imaginary worlds in varying proportions and be influenced or poorly interrogated. Their statements may be induced or suggested. A child may be sincere, convinced, and thus persuasive, and yet denounce fantasized abuse.

In France, we already knew what we pretend to discover today. Queen Marie-Antoinette wrote this to her sister Elisabeth from her cell at 4:30 AM on October 16, 1793, a few hours before her execution: "I have to speak to you about something very painful in my heart. I know how much grief this child must have caused you. Pardon him, my dear sister. Think of his age and how easy it is to make a child say what we want to hear, even what he does not understand."[13] Marie-Antoinette had been falsely accused of incest at her trial.

The role of the expert is to interpret and decipher the word of the child. What otherwise would be his mission? The literal interpretation of the narrative of the children in the Outreau case is not worthy of an expert. It led to erroneous conclusions and a judicial error that, were it not for the spectacular retraction of their mother, would have been upheld on appeal. In the assessment of the reliability of the revelation, the forensic analysis should never be limited to a word or drawing, be it troubling or distressing.

The Danger of Certainties

By eliminating doubt and alternative hypotheses, the militant approach, despite its noble intentions, seems to be more than simplistic; it is dangerous. The author believes that doubt, the ability to establish alternative hypotheses, and the willingness to provide the judge with a probabilistic approach and not a peremptory response are professional qualities in forensic expertise.

The peremptory style is even less acceptable where the opinion of the expert is founded on nonscientific arguments that are neither refutable nor verifiable. Such is the case with respect to the odd interpretation of drawings and dreams. For example, the psychologist in the Outreau case recalled in his report the shrew with a big tail in a drawing by one of the children subject to an expert assessment.[14] Also, a psychologist unfortunately appointed in the Outreau case as an expert had already acted ruthlessly in several other incest cases. Regarding a father accused of incest who had shared his nightmares with him since his detention, the expert stated: "His dreams point toward his guilt without the possibility of challenging this interpretation."

It may be difficult for our American colleagues to imagine that French judges would give any credit to such expert assessments. However, it is a reality. No one is a winner: neither justice nor the persons being tried, and even less so the search for truth. Since the Outreau case, noticeable changes were made. Experts are no longer granted life terms but are appointed for a period of 5 years. Throughout their entire career, they must certify as to all training taken. However, in-depth discussion must be pursued in particular with respect to expert methodology. The expert must no longer convey his feelings to the judge, but should provide a true analysis based on scientific literature, verifiable or refutable by his peers.

Analysis of the Reliability of a Revelation

The analysis of a revelation or a disclosure of abuse is of such complexity that it should never be limited to a single word, drawing, or symptom. Each expert assessment should contain a chapter titled *The Revelation* with a retrospective analysis of the conditions in which the revelation was made. This analysis should always succinctly include the following components, whether the child makes a direct denunciation or the family entourage is at the origin of the report:

- The personality and history (psychiatric, medical, and legal) of the alleged abuser
- The personality and history of the nonabusing or protective parent
- The nature of the first revelation, reported as literally as possible if the revelation was verbal or described precisely if the revelation was nonverbal
- The context of the first revelation (eg, whether it was spontaneous or made in response to questions, and if so, which questions in particular)
- The broader socioenvironmental circumstances in which the revelation occurred (eg, dynamics of parental separation if applicable, history of suspicions, the emotional character of the event, and psychofamilial issues)
- The assessment of the alleged victim (eg, physical or behavioral consequences, psychomotor development, history of truthfulness, quality of relationship with each parent).

Such analysis ensures that all focus is not simply on the content of the revelation and helps to cool down the debate, but remains vigilant with respect to the context of the revelation and the dynamics of the family.

THE TRIAL AS A FORM OF THERAPY

The therapeutic virtues of the criminal trial, perceived as a prerequisite to providing psychological remedies to victims, have often been highlighted by French psychologists. Many lawyers representing civil parties have often placed a responsibility on judges that should never have been there in the first place in arguing that acquitting the accused is, in some ways, tantamount to removing from the victim all hope of curing his or her traumatism. Criminal lawyers know that the public rarely identifies with the criminal in the box and that the compassion that the victim arouses, even more so in the case of a child, is often a reflection of its loathing for the accused. We have seen that it is assumed that the child speaks the truth; a child rarely lies, and any attempt to elicit such argument in court is dangerous.

Special Statutory Limits

Similar arguments were presented with respect to convincing the legislature to extend the limitation period for public actions. In France, this period has been extended to 20 years after the age of majority (ie, the age of 38 years). For childhood victims, there is consequently the issue of reliability with respect to memories of events in the past, which places experts in a difficult situation: how can one expect to truly illuminate the court with respect to events that occurred so long ago? The argument takes the form of a syllogism:

- It sometimes takes a whole life to make a revelation or disclose abuse
- A person cannot rebuild unless the abuse is acknowledged
- It is thus indispensable, when the alleged victim makes the revelation, that the court provides sanctions.

The nonapplication of statutory limits to sexual crimes and misdemeanors against minors is thus a recurring request of child protection agencies. Designating incest as the ultimate crime and denouncing the presumed complacency of the legislature in a "plea for the non-application of statutory limitation" that is as vibrant as it is demagogical, the psychiatrist and sexologist Philippe Brenot stated: "This hypocritical law prevents most women from reporting incest. Indeed, the very specific character of psychological development after incest has been ignored by the legislature unless it is a man participating in a collective denial of incest."[15]

Lack of Confrontation

The belief in the therapeutic virtues of a trial still occasionally leads judges, with the support of the experts, to eliminate decisive phases in the search for truth; this was shown in dramatic fashion in the Outreau case. Consequently, the filmed interviews of the Outreau children (which were mandatory pursuant to the law of June 17, 1998) were rare. It was said that video equipment was lacking and, during the investigation, the court did not want to inflict on the children conditions that would remind them of abuse, which had allegedly been filmed by their parents.

Similarly, no child in the Outreau case (including those who would later be found to be imaginary or fabricated victims) would be deemed to be able to attend a confrontation. The wording of the question posed to the experts was at least leading. The judge asked whether the confrontation was of a nature capable of reactivating the traumatism incurred by the children. The experts all responded in the affirmative even though confrontation is a fundamental right of the defense. Such methods are hard to accept and constitute a distortion of criminal justice. Strictly applying basic legal principles does not cause the victims additional pain but, on the contrary, guarantees to all the proper functioning of a constitutional government.

Confusion of Roles

The militant involvement of one of the female experts in the Outreau case, a psychologist but also the president of a child protection agency, raises another problem shown in these proceedings. What can be said about the attitude of an expert who confuses a trial with therapy and an investigation with treatment, thus offering the judges who trust them with a kind of all-in-one judicial proceeding? What can be said about an expert who speaks to the court of children subject to expert assessments as "her" children, for which she claims to be the maternal substitute? Can a forensic expert assessment be conducted with a bleeding heart overcome with passion and even fantasy? Can the story provided by a child alleged to be a victim be objectively examined if one confuses psychological and judicial remedies determining that one remedy must be given priority with respect to the other?

The ethics of experts prohibit them from conducting expert assessments in cases in which they were the therapist of the patient. The bitter lesson inflicted on our colleague in Saint-Omer, evicted from the courtroom during the trial, shows that the reverse should be true: All experts should refrain from providing therapy to individuals who are examined in connection with an expert assessment. Failing to exclude such a possibility as a matter of principle results, in the long term, in confusing both missions (expert assessment and treatment) and affects the attitude of the expert-therapist. When these roles are confused, empathy overrides the clinical sense, and emotion abolishes distance and silences the critical sense. A commingling of feelings inevitably leads to a confusion of roles: the expert shamelessly replaces the investigators through the concept of credibility and assumes, by means of peremptory conclusions, a large part of the responsibility of the verdict. This confusion fails to serve justice, even when it is performed with the best intentions in the world.

BEYOND OUTREAU: WHAT NEEDS TO CHANGE?

The Outreau case was the most important case in France in the first part of this century. It featured a botched investigation seeking incriminating evidence with the accused imprisoned without reason for more than 2 years, a case with sudden developments and psychiatric and psychological experts held up to ridicule. Its consequences for the judicial system and the expert approach in France were significant but their effects have yet to be felt, and there is a risk that all has been forgotten.

Nothing will have changed after Outreau if we fail to conduct critical analyses of the conjunction of parameters and of the beliefs or passions established as dogma that permitted such a shipwreck. In the future, the accused persons will not be so lucky to have, as an accuser, a mythomaniac who retracts at the hearing; a militant expert, evicted during the course of the trial; or a mediatized court as ready to exonerate the accused as it is to tie them to a whipping post. If one continues to examine cases of child sexual abuse based on binary and overly simple criteria such as true/false, lies/truth, and limit the expert inquiry to the author/victim dyad, there will be little chance for durable and significant change in such cases.

For every Outreau case in the future, how many closed or secret trials will there be? How many improbable allegations will there be? How many verdicts issued for the benefit of the doubt based on the word of colleagues too peremptory in their judgment? In the Outreau case, the judge and expert also proved, in the most horrible fashion, that they could form a pathologic team.

At the author's examination in the appeal proceedings in the Outreau case, he had the opportunity to state that to condemn an innocent person, even to a light sentence, is to fabricate a victim. It also condemns the alleged victim to live with this status for life, which is tragic if the abuse never occurred. A true discussion must now be engaged. Unfortunately, it took a shipwreck to be heard.

Limits of Expertise

The most lasting lesson does not concern the word of the child. Even today, only in exceptional circumstances will an expert challenge the veracity of statements regarding abuse made by a child. What has been especially learned from the Outreau case is the limits of psychiatric and psychological expertise. Even the best among us can make mistakes. Further, the clinical hypotheses of the psychological or psychiatric expert must be taken for what they are: an attempt to find a psychological truth and in no way a means to establish a judicial truth in place of the judge or even less so a search for a historical truth. What truly occurred, sometimes many years before the revelation, in reality escapes all players involved in the trial. If experts are conscious of their own limits and the limits of science, they have fewer misgivings in offering the judge a prudent response: a probabilistic approach based on relevant methods recognized by their peers.

Validation by Peers

The Parliamentary Commission of Inquiry initially addressed the problem of counter-expertise or, in the event of refusal, the possibility of an expert assessment conducted by the defense. This occurrence remains rare in French courts with the so-called private expert assessment deemed to be partial if the expert is paid by the party requesting it. Our inquisitive criminal procedure system is thus diametrically opposed to Anglo-Saxon practices, and judicial experts, despite the occasional uncertain nature of their work, have authoritative power in the court room.

The discussion here must address an important question: how much longer can it be tolerated that psychiatric expert assessments take on the force or weight of a verdict? The era of the expert-sapiens who may not be contradicted in court must come to an end. Contradiction, assessment by peers, and diagnostic discussions respecting rules or courtesy and ethics are necessary changes in the search for truth. If court experts knew, in drafting or filing an assessment, that they would be subject to contradiction, they would undoubtedly be more prudent, rigorous, and methodological, which would be in the interests of all.

Sexual Exception

Can allegations of child sexual abuse be dealt with similarly to all allegations of other types of offenses? The answer is not clear. If the sexual exception is the rule, an experienced or competent judge is not needed to deal with the case. However, if child sexual abuse allegations are to be handled the same as all allegations of other types of offenses, judges will have to have a higher level of competency. The author's opinion is that allegations of child sexual abuse should indeed be treated like any other area in law. Regardless of whether the judge is starting a career or is near retirement, the key is to be competent. There is no valid reason for a judge to undermine the fundamental rights of the defense and to discard experts. Judges, lawyers, and experts all have important roles in the process.

Perhaps it is not possible and this sensitive field must remain a sexual exception in law because of the victim being a child, but, if so, this must be clearly stated. It must also be acknowledged that neither the collegiality nor the experience of judges or experts will fundamentally change this injustice.

SUMMARY

Psychiatric experts must not interfere in this debate between lawyers. They should at least refuse to support punitive measures without their knowledge. They must show courage in acknowledging that a revelation does not meet the reliability requirements established by scientific literature on this issue. This requirement is not tantamount to treating a child as a liar but simply reminds the judge that the word of the child may be influenced, solicited, or contaminated by the views of a close adult. Consequently, the legal examination of the word of the child requires a different level of prudence then during a visit with the psychotherapist: as in all areas of law, the accused must be given the benefit of the doubt. However, if psychiatric experts or psychologists make peremptory statements failing to raise any doubts they may have, then what chance will the accused have? Will experts not, on the pretext of protecting children, become prosecutors of sorts, providing scientific (or pseudoscientific) support to punitive measures by the courts? They should express their doubts (a professional quality in this field) and limits that are not only restricted to their knowledge but also to their art. In following this policy, the expert will never be dishonored and, even if sometimes tacitly invited, will avoid sitting in the chair of the judge.

ACKNOWLEDGMENTS

Dr Bensussan gratefully acknowledges the assistance of Marc di Ruggiero, a Canadian lawyer and member of the Bar of Ontario, in translating this article from French into English.

REFERENCES

1. Van Gijseghem H. *Expertise psychiatrique: Vérité psychique, vérité factuelle?* [Psychiatric expertise: Psychological truth, factual truth?] Colloque International, Le Malaise de L'Expert Psycho Juridique [International Symposium: The Uneasiness of Forensic Experts]. *Liège* (Belgium), November, 2002 [in French].
2. Bensussan P, Rault F. *La dictature de l'émotion: la protection de l'enfance et ses dérives.* [The dictatorship of emotion: child protection and its failures]. Paris: *Éditions Belfond*; 2002 [in French].
3. Devedjian P. *Outreau, le chantier de la procédure pénale.* [Outreau, criminal procedure under construction]. Le Figaro October 15, 2007 [in French].
4. Aubenas F. *La Méprise: L'Affaire d'Outreau.* [The error: the Outreau affair]. Paris: Seuil; 2005 [in French].
5. *Les experts en psychologie mis à la question par la Cour d'assises de Paris.* [Psychological experts questioned by the Criminal Court of Paris]. Le Monde November 19, 2005 [in French].
6. Bensussan P. *A perpétuité.* [Life sentence]. Le Monde December 6, 2005 [in French].
7. Hayez JY, Vervier JF, Charlier D. *De la crédibilité des allégations des mineurs d'âge en matière d'abus sexuel.* [The credibility of allegations of minors in cases of sexual abuse]. *Psychiatrie de l'enfant* 1994;37(2):361–94 [in French].
8. Gabarini L, Petitot F. *La fabrique de l'enfant maltraité.* [The fabric of child abuse]. Toulouse (France): *Éditions Eres*; 1998 [in French].
9. Balzac H. *Splendeurs et misères des courtisanes.* [Splendor and misery of courtisans]. Paris: Flammarion; 1847. [in French].
10. Van Gijseghem H. *L'enfant mis à nu, l'allégation d'abus sexuel, à la recherche de la vérité.* [The exposed child, the allegation of sexual abuse, search for truth]. Montreal (Canada): *Editions du Méridien*; 1992 [in French].
11. Olivier-Gaillard C. *Processus de contamination par l'interrogatoire.* [Process of contamination by questioning]. Pratiques Psychologiques 2000;4:33–47 [in French].
12. Television show: *Mots croisés* (Crosswords). France 2, January 21, 2002.
13. Testament of Marie-Antoinette. October 16, 1793. Available at: http://www.histoire-de-france-et-d-ailleurs.com/articles/Testaments/TestamentMarieAntoinette.htm. Accessed November 6, 2010.
14. Leprêtre E. Psychological expert report of Mr Paul Gheyssens. June 14, 2000.
15. Brenot P. *De l'évitement naturel à l'imprescriptibilité de l'inceste.* [From natural avoidance to the non-application of statutory limitation in cases of incest]. Synapse 2003;194:15–8 [in French].

On the Use and Misuse of Genomic and Neuroimaging Science in Forensic Psychiatry: Current Roles and Future Directions

Michael T. Treadway, MA[a],*, Joshua W. Buckholtz, PhD[a,b,c],*

KEYWORDS

• Neuroimaging • Genetics • Law • Forensic assessment
• MAOA • Legally relevant psychopathology

With rapid advances having been made across multiple levels of genetic, molecular, and cognitive neuroscience, new questions arise as to when, whether, and how this enhanced knowledge of the neurobiological basis of human behavior will affect social institutions such as the criminal justice system. While some of these questions have focused on the potential uses of neuroimaging for lie detection and other forms of mind reading, an additional point of intersection between law and neuroscience resides in forensic psychiatry. As in other areas of psychiatry, the enhanced understanding of brain function offered by novel in vivo imaging technologies holds great promise for improved reliability and validity in diagnosis and assessment. Although we are cautiously optimistic about the longer-term benefits that may accrue from the introduction of neuroscience into the courtroom, the current tools have significant limitations. These caveats must be weighed heavily given the potential of neuroscientific data to

This manuscript work was produced with the support of the National Institute of Mental Health (F31MH087015) to M.T.T. and (T32MH018921) to J.W.B.
[a] Department of Psychology, Vanderbilt University, 301 Wilson Hall, Nashville, TN 37203, USA
[b] Vanderbilt Brain Institute, Vanderbilt University, Nashville, TN, USA
[c] Department of Psychology, Harvard University, Northwest Science Building - East Wing, Room 295.01, 52 Oxford Street, Cambridge, MA 02138, USA
* Corresponding author. Department of Psychology, Vanderbilt University, 301 Wilson Hall, Nashville, TN 37203; Department of Psychology, Harvard University, Northwest Science Building - East Wing, Room 295.01, 52 Oxford Street, Cambridge, MA 02138.
E-mail addresses: m.treadway@vanderbilt.edu; joshua.buckholtz@vanderbilt.edu

Child Adolesc Psychiatric Clin N Am 20 (2011) 533–546
doi:10.1016/j.chc.2011.03.012
1056-4993/11/$ – see front matter © 2011 Elsevier Inc. All rights reserved.

hold significant prejudicial, and at times, dubious probative, value for addressing questions relevant to criminal responsibility and sentencing mitigation.[1,2]

This article therefore summarizes, based on the current state of the science, the informational value provided to forensic psychiatry by two key neuroscientific domains with potential relevance to law: neuroimaging and genetics. This article is not intended to be comprehensive in terms of all possible uses of these technologies in any legal context, but rather limits its focus to forensic practice as it relates to the determination of insanity, diminished capacity, and mitigation. The first section reviews the current state of behavioral genetic research as it pertains to what is hereafter termed "legally relevant psychopathology" (LRP); that is, personality traits, behaviors, and diagnoses that may affect such forensic assessments (eg, impulsivity, substance abuse, antisocial personality disorder). The second section reviews basic principles of widely available neuroimaging tools and highlights some of the conceptual and analytical challenges of using these instruments to aid forensic assessment. Finally, in the third section, the authors look toward the future to identify certain trends that may overcome the limitations described in the preceding 2 sections.

FORENSIC GENETICS

On the occasion of the first draft release of the human genome, the full complement of inherited material possessed by the humans, Francis Collins (then the Head of the National Human Genome Research Institute) remarked, "What more powerful form of study of mankind could there be than to read our own instruction book." Although Collins likely intended this as a general comment on the utility of genetic information for understanding our evolutionary history and shared biology, this statement perhaps encapsulates a sentiment (or hope) that is increasingly held by many in the field of law: that analyzing an individual's DNA sequence can resolve the mystery of that individual's past and future behavior. However, whereas technological innovations of the last quarter century have rendered the human genome accessible to scientific inquiry in ways never before thought possible, the ethical, legal, and social implications of the resulting flood of genetic information are far from settled. With respect to the law, interest in the use of genetic information in the courtroom is often centered on two components of forensic psychiatry. First, criminal responsibility, that is, whether or not the genetic makeup of an individual influenced their behavior in such a way as to diminish their level of moral responsibility for a given criminal act, thereby mitigating their criminal liability; and sceond, criminal prediction, the extent to which information about the genetic makeup of an individual can be useful for determining that individual's future propensity toward criminality. Although a comprehensive and nuanced discussion of the implications of recent genetic discoveries for specific criminal contexts is beyond our expertise, we highlight several general issues pertaining to human behavioral genetics as a way of setting expectations for what is reasonable for legal thinkers to expect from genetics based on the state of the science.

In weighing the utility of genetic information for the determination of criminal responsibility and risk, it is instructive to contrast the goals of science with the goals of law. Scientific advances often proceed by use of inductive logic, whereby general conclusions are drawn from a collection of individual observations. For example, in genetic association studies, individuals with a certain genotype are grouped together and the frequency of a trait, behavior, or disorder is compared between the genotype groups. A statistically significant difference in the occurrence of that trait, behavior, or disorder between the two genotype groups is taken as an evidence of a positive genetic association. The strength of that association can be considered in terms of (as one example) an odds ratio, in which a "risk" genotype is considered to confer a certain degree of increased susceptibility to that trait, behavior, or disorder, relative to the "nonrisk" genotype. This way, a general phenomenon is derived by averaging across multiple single data points—that is, we are "inferring up" from the specific to the general. However, there may be many individuals (depending on the strength of the association) who possess the "risk" genotype, yet are completely psychiatrically healthy. In contrast, the application of genetics in forensic and legal settings depends on a process of "inferring down" to a specific individual's mental status on the basis of group-level phenomena, such as prior statistically significant genetic associations. Several examples are included in the following sections to demonstrate the difficulties inherent to this approach.

First, let us consider the concept of heritability. It has been understood since ancient times that certain forensically relevant traits and behaviors (eg, antisocial behavior and aggression) seem to run in families. Indeed, the apparent inheritance of such traits and behaviors has piqued the interest of modern science, and the question of their heritability has been a major target of scientific investigation. Heritability refers to the proportion of population variance in a trait or behavior that is accounted for by genetic factors, and is commonly measured by comparing the degree to which a trait or behavior is shared between dizygotic and monozygotic twins. Importantly, heritability in this context has a very specific meaning: because heritability deals with how much of the variability across a large number of people can be attributed to genetic factors, the concept of heritability bears little relevance for the individual person. For example, multiple genetic studies of antisociality converge to suggest that genetic factors account for approximately half of the population variability in antisocial traits and behaviors.[3] This does not mean that, in a given antisocial individual, half of his or her behavior is due to his or her genes and the other half to his or her environment. Herein lies the problem in inferring down from heritability. Even given the knowledge that genetic factors play a large role in an LRP, and given the understanding that, for whatever legal reason, the presence or absence of genetic factors is relevant for a specific individual determination of criminal responsibility or risk, it is impossible to know whether, in a specific individual, genetic factors play any role whatsoever in the presenting clinical phenomenon.

Thus, the mere knowledge that a given (putatively) legally relevant psychiatric phenomenon is heritable is not useful from a legal standpoint because heritability does not provide information about genetic contributions to the behavior of any one individual. However, knowing that a trait or behavior is heritable is useful insofar as it represents an essential starting point for further genetic analysis. Given heritability, the next step is to identify specific inherited genetic variants and mutations that are responsible for the intergenerational transmission of a trait, behavior, or disease.

It should be recalled that genes provide instructions for making proteins. According to the traditional genetic dogma one gene directs the creation of one protein (although it is now known that a single gene can code for a multitude of distinct, but related, proteins), and this information is stored as a four-letter DNA code. These letters are the DNA base pairs (bp): A (adenine), T (thymine), G (guanine), and C (cytosine), and the specific sequence in which these letters are arrayed within a gene determines the composition and abundance of the resulting protein. In humans, approximately 99% of this sequence is shared across members of our species, and it is thought that the 1% that varies between individuals is incredibly important for determining individual differences in traits ranging from eye color and height to one's predisposition for developing a range of physical and mental illnesses.

Some traits and diseases are known to result, deterministically, from a single well-characterized mutation or set of mutations within a single gene. For example, sickle cell disease is caused by a single mutation, the substitution of an "A" with a "T" at a specific position in the DNA sequence of the hemolgobin-β (HBB) gene, which leads to a detrimental change in the function of the oxygen transport protein hemoglobin. Individuals who possess 2 copies of this mutation (ie, one from each parent) develop the disease with 100% certainty. Thus, the presence or absence of the mutated "T" allele determines the presence or absence of the disease, and knowing whether an "A" or a "T" is present at that specific place in the DNA sequence of the HBB gene conveys, with complete fidelity, information about the disease state of the individual. In such so-called monogenic or mendelian disorders, the heritability of disease (or, as is the case, trait, or behavior) can be traced clearly to the inheritance of the mutation within affected families.

It is taken for granted that genetic information pertaining to these types of monogenic disorders (eg, Down syndrome, fragile X, Huntington disease) can be of value in circumstances that require specific evidence to confirm the presence of an organic disorder leading to mental impairment. However, in the case of most of the traits, behaviors, and disorders that are relevant to law, mendelian inheritance is the exception, rather than the rule. Indeed, the genetic architecture of psychopathology that is potentially relevant to the law (eg, substance abuse, antisocial behavior, psychosis) is polygenic and multifactorial, with common polymorphic variants in multiple genes, each of small effect size, interacting with each other and with the individual environment to predispose the risk for psychopathology.[4] Therefore, given the genetic complexity of these disorders, it becomes meaningless to talk about, much less, test an individual for, a "gene for" violence or a "gene for" addiction (to give but two examples). Instead, we infer a causal (but, critically, nondeterministic) relationship between one or more variants and a disease, behavior, or trait, on the basis of a statistical analysis of the frequency of that variant in people who possess that disease, behavior, trait and in those who do not. Typically, this analysis is accomplished by comparing the distribution of alleles at one or more polymorphic sites within a given gene's DNA sequence between individuals with or without a disorder. If 1 allele is found to be "overrepresented" in ill individuals (ie, found more commonly in people with illness than would be expected by chance), it can be said that this allele is associated with the disease and an odds ratio can be computed to quantify the degree of increased risk for the disease conferred by possessing the overrepresented allele. Similar methods can be used to quantify the degree of variance in a continuous trait (eg, scores on personality tests measuring impulsivity and aggression) accounted for by a given genetic variant.

The genetic complexity of LRPs requires that genetic associations to an LRP be considered as evidence that risk-associated genetic variants increase susceptibility to an LRP in a nondeterministic manner. Testing an individual for an allele that has been previously statistically associated with an LRP provides low-fidelity information about the presence or absence of that LRP in the individual. Further, in a given individual with a clinically diagnosed LRP, it is impossible to determine, even if they do possess a risk-associated allele, whether possessing that allele is in any way relevant to their psychiatric status because such "risk" alleles are, considered in isolation, completely compatible with psychiatric health. Consistent with this notion, effect sizes for the genetic variants that have been most consistently associated with LRPs (eg, antisocial behavior) are typically small,[4] commonly with odds ratios of less than 2, and often less than 5% of the variability in risk for a given trait, behavior, or disorder accounted for by a single genetic marker.[5] Furthermore, nonreplications of single genetic variants to clinical diagnostic phenotypes are common. To exemplify these issues, we consider the genetic factor that is most commonly considered with respect to LRPs, a polymorphic variant in the monoamine oxidase A (MAOA) gene.

MAOA encodes the mitochondrial catabolic enzyme monoamine oxidase A (MAO-A), which is important for degrading monoamine neurotransmitters such as serotonin.[6] Both human and animal studies point to a functional role for MAO-A in impulsive-aggressive behavior. For example, in a landmark article, Brunner and colleagues[7] examined a large Dutch kindred that was notorious for the high levels of impulsive and violent behavior demonstrated by some of its males. The character-istic behavioral phenotype, which stretched back for many generations, included mild mental retardation; extreme reactive aggression; and violent criminal behavior, including rape, assault and attempted murder, arson, and exhibitionism.[7] Affected males showed altered serotonin metabolism,[8,9] and females in this family were asymptomatic, which suggested that the heritable factor was located on the X chromosome.[7] Indeed, subsequent genetic analysis revealed the cause to be a point mutation (C936T) in the eighth exon of the X-linked MAOA gene. This mutation, which was present in all affected individuals, results in a premature stop codon. Thus, males who possess this mutation (and who have only one X chromosome) can be considered to have a functional knockout of their MAOA gene.[9]

We detail the Brunner finding of a highly functional but exceedingly rare mutation (it is not found outside of that one family) to contrast it with a polymorphic variant in the MAOA gene that has generated much interest for both psychiatry and law. In 1998, Sabol and colleagues[10] described a common, likely functional, so-called variable number of tandem repeats (VNTR) polymorphism in the upstream region of the MAOA gene. The MAOA u-VNTR (as it is sometimes called), is comprised of a repeated sequence of 30 bp; in vitro studies have shown that the presence of 3.5 or 4 repeats is associated with relatively higher MAOA expression (and are thus referred to as MAOA-H alleles), whereas the presence of 3 repeats results in relatively lower expression (MAOA-L allele).[10,11] Thus, by extension, individuals who possess 3.5 or 4 repeats of the 30-bp sequence have higher levels of MAOA (and therefore lower levels of sero-tonin) and individuals who possess 3 repeats of the 30-bp sequence have lower levels of MAOA (and therefore higher levels of serotonin). However, the functional signifi-cance of this variant in vivo has been called into question: one recent positron emis-sion tomographic (PET) study showed no effect of this variant on MAOA protein levels in the living human brain.[12]

The discovery of the MAOA u-VNTR was greeted with great enthusiasm by psychi-atric geneticists, who immediately began the search for associations of this variant to behavior and temperament. Given the linking of altered MAOA function to antisocial behavior by Brunner and colleagues,[7] special emphasis was placed on finding asso-ciations to manifest behavior and to traits that are empirically and conceptually related to aggression and impulsivity. Several behavioral instruments, diagnostic measures, and temperament indices have been used to test for an association between the MAOA-L allele and LRPs, including the Diagnostic and Statistical Manual of Mental Disorders (Fourth Edition) diagnoses of antisocial personality disorder (in adults), conduct disorder (in children and adolescents), and impulsive-antisocial traits as measured by the Tridimensional Personality Questionnaire, Temperament and Character Inventory, and NEO-Personality Inventory-Revised (NEO-PI-R).[13] Although some significant effects have been found, the size of such effects are typi-cally small (see earlier discussion); further, there are a number of nonreplications and prominent issues of allelic directionality (eg, associations of antisocial behavior to MAOA-H rather than to MAOA-L), which render interpretation difficult.[13,14] These conflicting findings, to date, are consistent with the idea that LRPs are both genetically and phenotypically complex. There are likely to be multiple genes that interact, with each other and with environmental factors (see later discussion), to affect the development of LRPs and further there may be distinct patterns of genetic linkages to relatively heterogenous subphenotypes within a broad diagnostic category (eg, distinct genetic architectures for reactive vs instrumental aggression within the broad diagnosis of antisocial personality disorder). On the whole, genetic studies of the *MAOA* u-VNTR support the notion that single common genetic variants, considered in isolation, provide little legally useful or relevant information for any given individual.

In contrast to the small and inconsistent effect of the *MAOA* u-VNTR on LRPs when considered as a single factor, there is evidence for a robust and replicable effect of this variant when the role of early life environment is taken into account. In a landmark study, Caspi and colleagues[15] found no effect of the MAOA u-VNTR on antisocial behavior on its own; however, a significant effect emerged in individuals who had experienced childhood maltreatment. This finding of a gene-environment interaction has been replicated (including via meta-analysis) and extended since the initial report.[16] However, in reflecting on the relevance of this finding for law, it is instructive to consider the data more closely. Specifically, these studies often find a significant primary effect for childhood maltreatment (but not *MAOA* u-VNTR genotype) on risk for adult antisocial behavior and aggression; stratifying individuals who experienced maltreatment by *MAOA* genotype reveals that the size of the effect of maltreatment on adult psychopathology is relatively stronger in MAOA-L individuals than in MAOA-H individuals. Two points are salient here: first, the primary risk factor for LRP is not a genetic factor (*MAOA* u-VNTR allele status) but an environmental one (childhood maltreatment) and second, the effect of this environmental factor is significantly weaker in individuals carrying an MAOA-H allele. Thus, it is entirely valid to think of the *MAOA* genotype as exerting a protective effect by buffering (in MAOA-H individuals) the otherwise adverse impact of childhood maltreatment.[17] Considered in this light, that is, the *MAOA*-H as protective allele rather than the *MAOA*-L as a liability allele, what is the legal relevance of *MAOA* genotype in an individual with a history of childhood abuse? From the standpoint of determining criminal responsibility, is the absence of a protective factor completely equivalent to the presence of a liability factor?

The greatest challenge to the utility of genetic information in forensic settings is the fact that although a single genetic factor may confer a measurably increased risk for an LRP on average (ie, across a group of participants in one or more studies) it cannot be reasonably inferred that if present in any given individual on trial, this factor elevated, diminished, or in any way affected the risk for the particular individual. Consider one example: a defendant on trial for aggravated assault has a documented history of early life abuse, and genetic testing reveals that he possesses the 3-repeat allele of the 30-bp 5' upstream MAOA VNTR. Given that several prior studies have demonstrated that this combination results in a significantly increased odds ratio for aggressive or antisocial behavior,[15–17] it is understandably tempting for the defense to suggest that the defendant's genetic profile, together with his background, contributed to his behavior in ways that were beyond his control, thereby diminishing his responsibility. The problem with such an inference is that whereas this combination on average results in increased risk, this specific combination of factors in this specific individual may very well have no effect on his antisocial behavior. This kind of inference ignores a myriad other factors that may exert a tremendous influence on the relationship between the specific measured variable that is associated, at the population level, with an LRP, and with behavior in that individual. In particular, this inference ignores the critical role of epistasis. Although only 1 genetic variant may be measured at a time, genetic variants do not exist in isolation to produce effects on brain and behavior. Rather, they exist as part of a complex and interacting network of genetic variation. It is increasingly understood in psychiatric genetics that epistatic interactions between variants can produce effects that would not necessarily be predicted on the basis of the main effects of the variants in isolation.[18–20] Thus, measuring 1 variant in isolation and making inferences about the causal role of that variant on an LRP can be misleading because, depending on an individual's larger genetic background, that variant, in that individual, may have either no effect or the opposite effect from what would be predicted on the basis of group-averaged population studies. Without being able to evaluate the full range of possible genetic and environmental factors that may increase, diminish, or nullify the effect of a particular genetic marker, it is challenging to infer accurately how much of an influence such a marker might have had for a particular individual on that particular individual's LRP.

On the whole, given the issues outlined earlier, it can be concluded that there are significant limitations with respect to the ability of genetic information to add value in addressing forensic questions pertaining to criminal responsibility, excepting of course cases in which the genetic diagnosis of simple, monogenic disorders is relevant to a particular case. However, we believe that these limitations are not necessarily insuperable. We do not wish to imply that the genetics of complex traits and disorders will never have a place in the courtroom, only that the present state of the science is such that the kind of genetic information currently available (or at least, most commonly offered in court) does not carry robust and reliable information about the cognitive capacities and mental state of an individual above and beyond what can be gleaned from clinical interviews and neuropsychological testing.

FORENSIC NEUROIMAGING

As with genetics, significant excitement has been generated by the possible application of neuroimaging in the courtroom, with proposed uses ranging from lie detection[21–24] and assessment of *mens rea*[25] to assessment of personality traits and diagnosis of LRP. The term neuroimaging encompasses a wide range of in vivo measurement techniques that may be used to capture different indices of brain structure and function. In humans, the most commonly used neuroimaging methods include electroencephalography (EEG), positron emission tomography (PET), single-photon emission computed tomography (SPECT), computed tomography (CT), and magnetic resonance imaging (MRI). As a class, these tools are thought to hold great promise in the advancement of medical diagnosis and the prediction of human behavior.[26]

Neuroimaging is advantageous because it is relatively accessible, noninvasive, and shows high reliability.[27] In a forensic context, use of neuroimaging may eventually be able to provide empirical evidence for the presence of an LRP, such as schizophrenia, which would be relevant in determining a defendant's capacity to have formulated criminal intent at the time of a crime. Similarly, neuroimaging evidence could theoretically provide compelling data to suggest impairment in neural processes required for cognitive control over impulsive behavior, which might aid a defendant seeking to plead down from a first- to a second-degree murder charge.

However, the current level of applicability of these techniques to the identification of LRP varies significantly. As stated earlier, the application of neuroimaging within the context of the courtroom hinges on the ability to infer down to the level of the individual. For reasons that are discussed later, many of the most widely publicized forms of neuroimaging (eg, functional MRI [fMRI]) are poorly suited for drawing inferences about the brain status of a specific individual. This section provides a brief review of the methodologies involved in these techniques, with a particular focus of how the interpretation of their results may be influenced by field-specific jargon that could increase their prejudicial value in a courtroom context. Finally, the strengths and weaknesses of different imaging techniques within the context of forensic assessment for LRP are reviewed.

Neuroimaging for the Assessment of Brain Abnormalities

In considering the application of neuroimaging data to forensic assessment, a distinction must be drawn between whether the neuroimaging data are to be used for demonstrating the presence of brain abnormalities (in the form of congenital malformations, significant atrophy, or traumatic insults resulting from injury, stroke, etc) or for the direct assessment of an LRP. Arguably, the most straightforward and noncontroversial applications of neuroimaging data are in cases of the former, in which such data simply provide confirmation that a given individual has experienced some sort of brain damage. This function is primarily accomplished through the use of structural neuroimaging, including CT and structural MRI scans, both of which provide excellent means of assessing the presence or absence of gross morphologic abnormalities on an individual basis. However, simply determining that damage is present says little regarding the implications of such damage for criminal behavior. The use of neuroimaging for this purpose makes no attempt to form a direct link between the mere presence of brain damage and LRP. Rather, this gap is bridged by the standard forms of neuropsychological assessment that seek to reveal specific cognitive and behavioral impairments that have more direct relevance for a client's actions, for which neuroimaging data merely serve as context or precondition. For example, in the well-publicized case of Terry Schiavo, both EEG and CT images were presented to demonstrate the extent of brain atrophy that had occurred. However, the interpretation of this data regarding the diagnosis of a persistent vegetative state relied on the testimony of several expert witnesses in neurology and neuropsychology, not the neuroimaging data itself.[28] Similarly, in the case of an insanity defense, neuroimaging can be used to establish that an individual's brain has experienced some form of damage, but its utility for assessing whether an individual was able to know the difference between right and wrong at the time of the crime is not yet known.

Neuroimaging for the Assessment of an LRP

In contrast to addressing questions regarding the presence of brain abnormalities that may buttress the use of neuropsychological assessment, some scientists and legal experts have increasingly promulgated neuroimaging as an alternative, and more powerful, means of directly measuring LRP. In the eyes of its proponents, neuroimaging techniques hold the promise to catch the predispositions toward impulsivity, poor cognitive control, and the like that the current battery of assessment instruments fail to capture. Speculation on this second use of neuroimaging data in criminal law has generated equal enthusiasm and criticism among scholars and commentators, although at present, there are few examples from which to draw concrete information on how such data might be used in the courtroom.

To make claims that the presence of a brain abnormality may result in an LRP, it must be shown that either prior data has specifically linked the same abnormality to the same legally-relevant impairment, or there is sound reason to believe that the abnormality could produce such an impairment, given what is generally known about its role or function. In both cases, information about typical brain function (as derived from group studies) must be inferred down to the individual level. However, as demonstrated in the discussion later, data reduction and analysis methods common to almost all neuroimaging techniques may significantly compromise the ability of these techniques to provide accurate or meaningful information about a specific person. The following sections, highlight specific steps in the analysis of imaging datasets that are most problematic for the purposes of individual prediction.

Normalization of Brain Images

Although the macro architecture of the human brain is shared across individuals, each person's brain shows variation in both subtle and gross morphologic aspects. Consequently, studies that seek to identify common loci of neurobiological processes using standard noninvasive brain imaging techniques are required to find ways to bring each individual brain into a "common space." Referred to as "normalization," this process uses a series of iterative algorithms to transform the data of each subject to match the spatial properties of a group average template. For the purposes of group analysis, it is reasonable to assume that errors in normalization will be randomly distributed, and will therefore cancel each other out when looking at group-averaged data. However, this assumption does not apply when trying to draw inferences from a particular individual. Consider an example in which a region of interest (ROI) for a specific neuroimaging task is the dorsal portion of the anterior cingulate cortex, which is known to exhibit several common sulcal variations.[29,30] What inferences could be drawn if no activation was shown in the area of anterior cingulate most commonly found in group studies but was present in a neighboring region? Such a pattern could suggest an impairment in the dorsal cingulate function that might be of relevance, or merely a normalization error reflecting a typical structural variation in the cingulate morphology for the individual in question.

Voxelwise Statistical Inference

All functional neuroimaging datasets divide the brain into 3-dimensional pixels, or voxels. Voxels are typically 3 to 4 mm^3, but may get smaller than 1 mm^3 when using particularly high-field strength magnets (eg, 7 Tesla strength or higher). Analysis of these voxels is typically performed on a per-voxel basis. That is, if the brain is divided into n voxels, the analysis will require n number of individual statistical tests. However, neither neuroimaging data nor the neural events are independent to the extent that would be necessary for voxelwise approaches to represent an ideal analytical technique. Increasing evidence suggests the presence of multiple state-dependent neural networks that are highly intercorrelated.[31] Moreover, sources of noise from MRI and PET imaging techniques are also correlated, despite sophisticated filtering techniques used to reduce their influence. The consequence is a reduced statistical power to detect real effects, leading to a high degree of type II error across many neuroimaging studies.[32] This elevated rate of false negatives, although still problematic in group studies, is a far more serious problem when attempting to assess data from a single individual when attempting to draw an inference about the presence or absence of an LRP.

Linking Neuroimaging Data to Brain States: Problems of Interpretation

Functional neuroimaging, be it through EEG, PET, SPECT or fMRI, provides an indirect measure of neuronal information processing. Of these measures, only EEG directly assesses the electric activity of neurons, although it is limited in its ability to accurately represent specific regions from which electric signals emanate. The other 3 techniques provide measures of cellular metabolism. Because neuronal activity, including both the generation of an action potential ("firing") as well as the processing of received impulses from other neurons, is energetically demanding, isolating changes in metabolic activity may serve as a useful index for the engagement of neurons. Within the neuroimaging research literature, this type of engagement is often referred to as "activation." The term activation may be misleading, however, because it is really a nonspecific index of some form of neuronal process, which may range from a neuron firing to a neuron increasing the expression of a particular gene to a neuron entering a depolarized state (ie, becoming less likely to fire).[33] Consequently, although these measures may be used to identify general brain regions in which changes in metabolic activity are associated with completion of a specific behavioral task the functional significance of this change in metabolism is unknown.

In addition to the potentially misleading nature of terms such as "activation," another often-underappreciated aspect of fMRI is that it is highly state dependent. That is to say, there exists no baseline for brain activity; only relative changes in activity during an experimental condition as compared to a relevant control condition. Consider an example of an individual who is being charged for a crime involving an impulsive act of violence. His defense team has already shown that he performs poorly on cognitive tests that asses an individual's ability to inhibit a prepotent response, such as the go/no-go or stop-signal task, and they hope to sway the court further by showing that when performing these tasks in the scanner, his brain shows altered responses in brain regions that have been demonstrated to underlie the performance of these tasks in group studies. The first question is what neuroimaging result would provide evidence for a legally-relevant brain impairment? Perhaps the first guess might be that an individual with impairment would show less "activation" in this region, as is consistent with many group case-control studies.[34–37] Although this is certainly a reasonable hypothesis, failure to detect signal in expected regions might simply reflect poor statistical power (as discussed earlier). Alternatively, other case-control studies have suggested that impaired performance may manifest as greater "activation," indicating a neural network inefficiency.[38,39] For this latter interpretation, it is hypothesized that if the first group shows greater activation in a brain region to achieve the same level of performance as a second group, the activation of the first group is said to be less efficient than that of the second. Consequently, we are left with 2 plausible hypotheses for why more- or less-than-expected activity might reflect a functional impairment.

Taken together, technical limitations in neuroimaging analysis and interpretation significantly curtail the incremental value of these techniques in the assessment of LRP over the standard neuropsychological measures. These limitations include the problem of group versus individual brain morphology, the low statistical power of many neuroimaging studies, unanswered questions regarding the appropriate physiologic interpretation of functional neuroimaging data, and a lack of hypotheses that may definitively distinguish between the presence and absence of an LRP at the level of an individual.

FORENSIC NEUROSCIENCE IN THE NEXT DECADE

While this article has primarily focused on identifying limitations in the application of current genomic and neuroimaging technologies to forensic psychiatry, there have been recent developments in both areas that are likely to mitigate these limitations in the next 5 to 10 years. In this final section, we touch upon these promising advances.

Genetics

For genetics to be useful in forensic assessment, the field must move beyond a focus on single genetic variants in isolation to consider the impact of epistatic interactions between multiple genes on risk for LRPs, and between identified sets of multi-gene risk alleles and environmental influences. Multivariate datamining of large-scale prospective cohort designs will be important in determining the most robust, sensitive, and specific combination of genetic and environmental risk factors for use in legal settings. For example, a large sample longitudinal study that integrates detailed social, environmental, and mental health assessments with genome-wide sequencing, such as the recently launched National Child Study (www.nationalchildrensstudy.gov), can be interrogated with multivariate techniques to examine, in a data-driven manner, the precise combination of variables that is most predictive of LRPs. One question that will have to be decided by the courts, in consultation with neuroscience, is precisely how much of the variance in a specific LRP must be accounted for by such a combination of variables before it is considered relevant to the evaluation of criminal responsibility. We believe that a crucial next step for integrating genetic information into legal settings is the establishment of specific thresholds for the sensitivity, specificity, predictive utility of, and tolerance of subsequent nonreplication for, neurobiological measurements.

Neuroimaging

As stated earlier, although neuroimaging is clearly useful for the establishment of brain injury or trauma, its utility as a direct measure of LRP has yet to be established. However, recent breakthroughs in the analysis of neuroimaging datasets have emerged that may greatly enhance the ability to use these tools for individual diagnosis. A key advancement is the introduction of multivariate methods that use all the collected data points in a brain scan simultaneously, rather than treat them as individual voxels to be analyzed independently (as is typically done in current analytical methods). Consequently, concerns about warping, normalization, or differential recruitment of specific brain regions to perform a given task are ameliorated because interpretation of multivariate analysis is no longer constrained to a specific ROI.

Consistent with the idea that network-driven approaches show a greater power to provide neuroimaging-based assessments of LRP is their emerging success in diagnosing psychiatric and neurologic disorders. Within the last few years, both structural and functional neuroimaging data have been shown to accurately predict the onset of psychotic symptoms within a high-risk sample[40,41] and Alzheimer disease symptoms within a group of older individuals experiencing mild cognitive impairment.[42] In addition to prediction, these techniques have been increasingly shown to provide differential diagnosis, successfully discriminating between different mood disorders.[43] Finally, because multivariate techniques are able to integrate imaging and nonimaging data, a recent study found that the combination of neuroimaging and genetic data provided better accuracy for classification of individuals with schizophrenia than either technique alone.[44] Across these studies, the diagnostic accuracy rates have been as high as 85% to 90%, with sensitivity rates reaching more than 95%, indicating significant potential to improve on traditional clinician-based diagnostic methods.

Finally, public opinion is one other avenue through which neuroimaging and genetics may affect forensic psychiatry and the legal system generally. Current social institutions, including the law, explain human behavior through concepts of individual agency and free will, whereas these tools provide explanations that are purely mechanistic. As the ability to understand and predict the causes of behavior continues to accrue, it is possible that the public perception of what criminal responsibility is and how it should be punished will shift. Indeed, some legal experts have argued that it is in the domain of the legislature and public opinion that neuroscience will ultimately exert its greatest influence over the law, as opposed to the courtroom itself.[45]

SUMMARY

In this review, we have detailed the current obstacles to the use of genomic and neuro-imaging technologies to aid in forensic assessment, as well as discussed several recent developments that may help overcome these barriers. Although genomic and neuroimaging sciences are not yet making their impact felt on forensic practice, it seems likely that these technologies will increasingly play a role in the diagnosis of LRP.

REFERENCES

1. McCabe DP, Castel AD. Seeing is believing: the effect of brain images on judgments of scientific reasoning. Cognition 2008;107(1):343–52.
2. Weisberg DS, Keil FC, Goodstein J, et al. The seductive allure of neuroscience explanations. J Cogn Neurosci 2008;20(3):470–7.
3. Moffitt TE. Genetic and environmental influences on antisocial behaviors: evidence from behavioral-genetic research. Adv Genet 2005;55:41–104.
4. Meyer-Lindenberg A, Weinberger DR. Intermediate phenotypes and genetic mechanisms of psychiatric disorders. Nat Rev Neurosci 2006;7(10):818–27.
5. Burmeister M, McInnis MG, Zollner S. Psychiatric genetics: progress amid controversy. Nat Rev Genet 2008;9(7):527–40.
6. Shih JC, Chen K, Ridd MJ. Monoamine oxidase: from genes to behavior. Annu Rev Neurosci 1999;22:197–217.
7. Brunner HG, Nelen MR, van Zandvoort P, et al. X-linked borderline mental retardation with prominent behavioral disturbance: phenotype, genetic localization, and evidence for disturbed monoamine metabolism. Am J Hum Genet 1993; 52(6):1032–9.
8. Abeling NG, van Gennip AH, van Cruchten AG, et al. Monoamine oxidase A deficiency: biogenic amine metabolites in random urine samples. J Neural Transm Suppl 1998;52:9–15.
9. Brunner HG, Nelen M, Breakefield XO, et al. Abnormal behavior associated with a point mutation in the structural gene for monoamine oxidase A. Science 1993; 262(5133):578–80.
10. Sabol SZ, Hu S, Hamer D. A functional polymorphism in the monoamine oxidase A gene promoter. Hum Genet 1998;103(3):273–9.
11. Deckert J, Catalano M, Syagailo YV, et al. Excess of high activity monoamine oxidase A gene promoter alleles in female patients with panic disorder. Hum Mol Genet 1999;8(4):621–4.
12. Fowler JS, Alia-Klein N, Kriplani A, et al. Evidence that brain MAO A activity does not correspond to MAO A genotype in healthy male subjects. Biol Psychiatry 2007;62(4):355–8.
13. Buckholtz JW, Meyer-Lindenberg A. MAOA and the neurogenetic architecture of human aggression. Trends Neurosci 2008;31(3):120–9.
14. Buckholtz JW, Meyer-Lindenberg A. Gene-brain associations: the example of MAOA. In: Hodgins S, Viding E, editors. Persistent violent offenders: neuroscience and rehabilitation. Oxford (United Kingdom): Oxford University Press; 2009. p. 265–85.

15. Caspi A, McClay J, Moffitt TE, et al. Role of genotype in the cycle of violence in maltreated children. Science 2002;297(5582):851–4.
16. Kim-Cohen J, Caspi A, Taylor A, et al. MAOA, maltreatment, and gene-environment interaction predicting children's mental health: new evidence and a meta-analysis. Mol Psychiatry 2006;11(10):903–13.
17. Dodge KA. Mechanisms of gene-environment interaction effects in the development of conduct disorder. Perspect Psychol Sci 2009;4(4):408–14.
18. Nicodemus KK, Law AJ, Radulescu E, et al. Biological validation of increased schizophrenia risk with NRG1, ERBB4, and AKT1 epistasis via functional neuroimaging in healthy controls. Arch Gen Psychiatry 2010;67(10):991–1001.
19. Nicodemus KK, Callicott JH, Higier RG, et al. Evidence of statistical epistasis between DISC1, CIT and NDEL1 impacting risk for schizophrenia: biological validation with functional neuroimaging. Arch Gen Psychiatry 2010;67(10): 991–1001.
20. Pezawas L, Meyer-Lindenberg A, Goldman AL, et al. Evidence of biologic epistasis between BDNF and SLC6A4 and implications for depression. Mol Psychiatry 2008;13(7):709–16.
21. Davatzikos C, Ruparel K, Fan Y, et al. Classifying spatial patterns of brain activity with machine learning methods: application to lie detection. Neuroimage 2005; 28(3):663–8.
22. Langleben DD, Schroeder L, Maldjian JA, et al. Brain activity during simulated deception: an event-related functional magnetic resonance study. Neuroimage 2002;15(3):727–32.
23. Kozel FA, Revell LJ, Lorberbaum JP, et al. A pilot study of functional magnetic resonance imaging brain correlates of deception in healthy young men. J Neuropsychiatry Clin Neurosci 2004;16(3):295–305.
24. Kozel FA, Padgett TM, George MS. A replication study of the neural correlates of deception. Behav Neurosci 2004;118(4):852–6.
25. Brown T, Murphy E. Through a scanner darkly: functional neuroimaging as evidence of mens rea. Stanford Law Rev 2010;62:1119–208.
26. Singh I, Rose N. Biomarkers in psychiatry. Nature 2009;460(7252):202–7.
27. Poldrack RA, Mumford JA. Independence in ROI analysis: where is the voodoo? Soc Cogn Affect Neurosci 2009;4(2):208–13.
28. Perry JE, Churchill LR, Kirshner HS. The Terri Schiavo case: legal, ethical, and medical perspectives. Ann Intern Med 2005;143(10):744–8.
29. Leonard CM, Towler S, Welcome S, et al. Paracingulate asymmetry in anterior and midcingulate cortex: sex differences and the effect of measurement technique. Brain Struct Funct 2009;213(6):553–69.
30. Fornito A, Wood SJ, Whittle S, et al. Variability of the paracingulate sulcus and morphometry of the medial frontal cortex: associations with cortical thickness, surface area, volume, and sulcal depth. Hum Brain Mapp 2008;29(2): 222–36.
31. Huettel SA, Song AW, McCarthy G. Functional magnetic resonance imaging. 2nd edition. Sunderland (United Kingdom): Sinauer Associates, Inc; 2008.
32. Lieberman MD, Cunningham WA. Type I and Type II error concerns in fMRI research: re-balancing the scale. Soc Cogn Affect Neurosci 2009;4(4):423–8.
33. Logothetis NK. What we can do and what we cannot do with fMRI. Nature 2008; 453(7197):869–78.
34. Tanabe J, Tregellas JR, Dalwani M, et al. Medial orbitofrontal cortex gray matter is reduced in abstinent substance-dependent individuals. Biol Psychiatry 2009; 65(2):160–4.

35. Pizzagalli DA, Holmes AJ, Dillon DG, et al. Reduced caudate and nucleus accumbens response to rewards in unmedicated individuals with major depressive disorder. Am J Psychiatry 2009;166(6):702–10.
36. Smoski MJ, Felder J, Bizzell J, et al. fMRI of alterations in reward selection, anticipation, and feedback in major depressive disorder. J Affect Disord 2009;118: 69–78.
37. Koch K, Wagner G, Schultz C, et al. Altered error-related activity in patients with schizophrenia. Neuropsychologia 2009;47(13):2843–9.
38. Wagner G, Sinsel E, Sobanski T, et al. Cortical inefficiency in patients with unipolar depression: an event-related FMRI study with the Stroop task. Biol Psychiatry 2006;59(10):958–65.
39. Callicott JH, Mattay VS, Verchinski BA, et al. Complexity of prefrontal cortical dysfunction in schizophrenia: more than up or down. Am J Psychiatry 2003; 160(12):2209–15.
40. Sun D, van Erp TG, Thompson PM, et al. Elucidating a magnetic resonance imaging-based neuroanatomic biomarker for psychosis: classification analysis using probabilistic brain atlas and machine learning algorithms. Biol Psychiatry 2009;66(11):1055–60.
41. Koutsouleris N, Meisenzahl EM, Davatzikos C, et al. Use of neuroanatomical pattern classification to identify subjects in at-risk mental states of psychosis and predict disease transition. Arch Gen Psychiatry 2009;66(7):700–12.
42. Davatzikos C, Bhatt P, Shaw LM, et al. Prediction of MCI to AD conversion, via MRI, CSF biomarkers, and pattern classification. Neurobiol Aging Jun 29 2010. [Epub ahead of print].
43. Arribas J, Calhoun V, Adali T. Automatic Bayesian classification of healthy controls, bipolar disorder and schizophrenia using intrinsic connectivity maps from fMRI data. IEEE Trans Biomed Eng 2010;57:2850–60.
44. Yang H, Liu J, Sui J, et al. A hybrid machine learning method for fusing fMRI and genetic data: combining both improves classification of schizophrenia. Front Hum Neurosci 2010;4:192.
45. Maroney TA. The false promise of adolescent brain science in juvenile justice. Notre Dame Law Rev 2010;85:89.

Malingering in Children: Fibs and Faking

James S. Walker, PhD[a,b,c,*]

KEYWORDS

- Expert witness • Children and adolescents
- Forensic psychiatry • Forensic psychology • Malingering

Any parent is aware that a child can purposefully deceive others. It seems odd that there was controversy among psychologists and psychiatrists for a long time about whether children could malinger illness. Even more firmly ensconced among our profession was the thought that the clinician could always "just tell" when anyone, child or adult, was trying to purposefully feign an illness. Indeed, it required the groundbreaking set of studies by Faust and colleagues[1] to show that clinicians were susceptible to being misled, even by children.

In the first of those studies, neuropsychologists were given sets of cognitive test data produced by adolescents, aged 15 to 17 years, some of whom had been instructed to malinger and others not. The clinicians were asked to rate if they found the profiles to reflect pathology, and whether the results were attributable to brain injury, emotional factors, or malingering. In that study, 78% of the clinicians rated the profiles abnormal, but none of them attributed the findings to malingering. Moreover, 88% of the clinicians were at least moderately confident in their conclusions.

In a second study, the neuropsychologists were warned beforehand that there was a 50% malingering base rate among the subjects. Still, 91% of the neuropsychologists found the test results to be pathologic and 90% judged them to be valid. Their moderately confident or better ratings were 97%.

In the third study, children, aged 9 to 12 years, were asked to produce malingered neuropsychological test profiles. The clinicians were asked to rate if the profiles were organic, functional, or malingered. The neuropsychologists judged 93% of the profiles to be abnormal and 83% attributed the aberrant results to brain injury. None were identified as malingering. In 75% of the cases, the clinicians were moderately confident or better.

Dr Walker has nothing to disclose.
a Department of Psychology, Vanderbilt University, Nashville, TN, USA
b Private Practice of Neuropsychology, Nashville, TN, USA
c Neuropsychology Consultants, PLLC, 4219 Hillsboro Pike, Suite 203, Nashville, TN 37215, USA
* Neuropsychology Consultants, PLLC, 4219 Hillsboro Pike, Suite 203, Nashville, TN 37215.
E-mail address: jameswalker@neuroforensic.com

Child Adolesc Psychiatric Clin N Am 20 (2011) 547–556
doi:10.1016/j.chc.2011.03.013
childpsych.theclinics.com
1056-4993/11/$ – see front matter © 2011 Elsevier Inc. All rights reserved.

Although those studies were criticized on several grounds,[2] they awakened the profession of neuropsychology to the potential threat posed by poor effort or feigning of illness. Today, malingering is the most-researched topic in the field of neuropsychology. Even so, research regarding malingering by children lags far behind. This state of affairs probably reflects to some degree the lingering thoughts in psychiatry and psychology that children rarely malinger and, if they do, they are easily identified.

DECEPTION IN CHILDREN

Research shows that children regularly practice deceptive communication. There are reports in the literature of children as young as 21 months old deliberately prevaricating.[3] When left with a toy and told not to peek, 3-year-old peekers deny peeking 38% of the time.[4] The percentage of lying children seems to increase with age; 86% of 4- to 7-year-old children displaying similar behavior of denying transgressions, even though most of them are able to articulate the difference between truth telling and lying to the researchers.[5] Children as young as 9 years of age have been identified as sustaining malingering behavior in a traumatic brain injury case in which litigation was involved. That was conceptualized as a case of malingering by proxy in which the parents' motivations were critical in the child's behavior.[6] Adolescents can feign attention-deficit/hyperactivity disorder (ADHD) to obtain psychostimulant medication[7] and can easily simulate reports of ADHD symptoms.[8] Even children as young as 6 years of age are able to consistently underperform on cognitive testing when instructed to do so.[9]

CLINICAL VIGNETTES

Three illustrative examples from the author's practice show the potential for children to deceive or otherwise fake believable deficits.

Case 1
Amy was a 9-year-old third grader. Her father was an over-the-road trucker and her mother worked 2 jobs. Amy had 2 older brothers who were often left to care for her, but they paid little attention to her or her needs. One September morning during her first period at school, Amy announced to her teacher that her mother had died the night before. Her affect was bland when making this statement. The teacher, horrified, notified all of the other teachers and the principal. Amy was taken from class and went to the principal's office where she was lavished with concern and attention. Subsequent calls to her parents' home yielded no answers, but when one of her brothers at another school was contacted, he was bewildered and said that he was not aware of his mother's death. Further investigation revealed the mother to be alive, in good health, and at her usual place of employment. Subsequent psychotherapy showed Amy to be suffering from a significant degree of emotional neglect by her parents and caregivers. Indeed, to her, her mother had died, in that she was largely absent from her life. That was a pivotal event for the family and the mother decided to quit one of her jobs to spend more time with her children.

Case 2
Sam was an 11-year-old boy who developed boils on his lower body. These were large, swollen areas of infection that were excruciatingly painful and were accompanied by high fevers. The lesions were constantly present for a period of several weeks, with little improvement. When Sam was eventually taken to the pediatrician, he told the pediatrician that the lesions had been caused by the bites of a large orange insect he

had encountered in a walk through a field. Intrigued, being somewhat of an ento-mologist, the physician asked Sam to look through a pictorial index of insects. There, Sam identified a truly fearsome-looking orange beetle with a large, needle-shaped proboscis as his assailant. The description of this insect, however, indi-cated that it fed only on plants and flowers and was not venomous or dangerous to humans. When confronted with this information, the boy said that he had indeed come upon this insect in a walk through a field, but admitted that the story of the insect had been made up because he thought "it would be cool" for his illness to be caused by such a scary-looking creature. After being referred for psychotherapy, it was discovered that Sam was socially isolated because of his parents' intense reli-giosity and their fear of the larger culture. His father was an angry, brooding figure who was irritable, sharp tongued, and had little time to spend with his son. Sam had become immersed in his interests about insects, snakes, and other phenomena of nature to compensate for his lack of social adeptness. With therapy, over time he began to develop normal, age-appropriate friendships. His boils responded well to antibiotics.

Case 3

Derek was a 7-year-old boy who lived in public housing in inner-city Memphis with his mother and 6 siblings. His mother had a history of substance dependence and was not working. Three of his siblings were receiving supplemental security income (SSI) payments for various mental disorders, including mental retardation, depression, and disruptive behavior problems. When Derek's mother brought him to his own SSI evaluation for alleged disabilities of learning problems and ADHD, he behaved in an uncontrolled fashion in the waiting area. As soon as the examiner entered the waiting room, Derek began jumping up and down on the couch and slapping a nearby light fixture. His mother looked on calmly, making no attempt to corral her child or correct his behavior. Upon interview, during which the child roamed the office pulling out books, magazines, and files while his mother remained passive, she described a history of excessive activity and disruptive behavior. She produced a prescription for a stimulant medication written a few days before by the child's pediatrician. She said he was failing in school and had often been suspended. After the mother left the room, the child continued his disruptive behavior. However, he quickly ceased when asked to do so by the examiner. The examiner asked if anyone had asked him to say or do anything during his appointment that day. He replied that yes, his mother had told him to "act up" as much as possible or else the family would not be able to have enough money to buy food. A phone call to his teacher revealed that Derek was performing adequately in school, although he was struggling a bit with reading. His behavior at school was not a problem at all. He was rated as not having a significant mental impairment and the application for SSI disability benefits was denied.

These cases reflect the capacity of children to intentionally deceive others, although in each case the motivation was quite different. Only in the last case could the behavior be reasonably classified as malingering, yet in that case the child's only motivation was to follow his mother's instructions, a clear case of malingering by proxy. There was no conscious effort to deceive or a true appreciation on the child's part of the nature and context of the evaluation.

THE CLINICAL INTERVIEW AND HISTORY

As the case vignettes indicate, there is no substitute for the clinician's taking an active role in assessing for malingering behavior, even to the point of following up with collateral sources of information. There is also no substitute for the clinical interview. Although it has clearly been established that clinical evaluation alone is rarely sufficient for establishing the presence of malingering behavior, the information gained during the interview is critical for establishing the consistency of patients' symptom reports with other data.

Children, indeed, most patients, are at a disadvantage in attempting to malinger mental illness, because they rarely have a sufficiently sophisticated understanding of the presentation of the mental illness they hope to feign. Many malingering patients present with feigned syndromes based upon stereotypical ideas of mental illness, such as the child who has been disturbed since his grandfather died and has regular conversations with his ghost or the adolescent feigning mental retardation who appears in the clinician's waiting room clutching a stuffed animal and coloring book. Patients who report double vision with one eye covered or who describe whole-body convulsions with no loss of consciousness would immediately raise the suspicions of the astute clinician.

The mental status examination is also crucial. The tendency of malingerers to offer near-miss responses to simple questions, such as orientation (eg, date, day, year, location), is well known. Although normal patients often cannot recall more than 1 or 2 words after a few minutes, all but the most demented patients can accurately choose the words presented from a range of choices. Most persons with serious illness are to some degree embarrassed by their dysfunction and reluctant to discuss their symptoms, whereas malingerers often do so with relish. Also, malingerers often present with a hostile or noncompliant attitude, a most unusual style considering the potentially helpful nature of a mental health consultation. Malingerers often appear bewildered or look to a family member or companion for answers to overlearned personal information, such as marriage status, age, number and names of children, and so forth, while displaying a fair knowledge of recent, day-to-day information and events, a finding inconsistent with known memory syndromes.

The clinical interview also allows for an analysis of the consistency between patients' report of symptoms, their daily activities, observations of their abilities during the interview, their cognitive test results (if any), and reports from collateral sources. Analysis of such information is perhaps not sufficient, but is always helpful, in establishing the presence of malingering.[10,11]

FORMAL TESTS FOR MALINGERED PSYCHIATRIC SYMPTOMS
Self-Report Rating Scales

Many commonly used behavior rating scales for children, such as the Children's Depression Inventory[12] and the various forms of the Achenbach Child Behavior Checklist (CBCL),[13] lack any type of formal validity scales. This lack of validity is not to say that the test protocols cannot be examined by the clinician for consistency or potential exaggeration or used in conjunction with other data to aid in the assessment for malingering, but no data exists on the actual performance of malingerers on these tests as compared with genuine patients. Other behavior rating scales, such as the Trauma Symptom Checklist for Children,[14] have rudimentary validity scales for which little data exist regarding the performance of over-reporters.

The Behavior Assessment System for Children-2 (BASC-2) is currently the only comprehensive self-report measure for young children (<12 years of age) for which validity scales exist.[15] In a recent study (the only one of its kind[16]) children failing a test for cognitive malingering were also administered the BASC-2. Despite their failure of the cognitive malingering test, most of the children passed the validity scales of the BASC-2. This finding may demonstrate the relative insensitivity of the BASC-2 to malingering behavior in children or it may reflect the fact that children who are malingering memory problems may not always choose to also feign psychiatric or behavioral symptoms. To date, no data exist on the ability of the BASC-2 to distinguish simulators from genuine reporters, and the validation studies of the instrument neglected this critical procedure.

Self-Report Personality Inventories

The Minnesota Multiphasic Personality Inventory for Adolescents (MMPI-A) is the most widely used self-report scale for adolescents.[17] It contains variations of the same validity scales offered in the adult version of the instrument, but far less research data exist on the usefulness of the validity scales in identifying overreporters. In a group of adolescents, Rogers and his colleagues[18] found that the F scale (a scale measuring reporting of infrequent symptoms) was not as successful as the F minus K index (an index consisting of a scale measuring infrequent symptom report minus the score of a scale measuring socially desirable responding) in identifying overreporting adolescents. Other researchers reported good results using the F scale score alone.[19]

Another widely used personality inventory for adolescents is the Adolescent Psychopathology Scale.[20] This test was standardized on a large group of adolescents and contains an overreporting scale called Infrequency Response. Reynolds offers frequency data for clinical patients and their scores on this scale, but like the BASC-2 no simulation studies were performed in the development of this instrument and no research regarding the sensitivity of this scale has been performed to date. As a result, the clinician should interpret the results of this test with caution.

Third-Party Rating Scales

Many clinicians rely upon the ratings of third parties, usually parents and teachers, in the assessment of preadolescent children. The previously mentioned Child Behavior Checklist and the BASC-2 each offer versions for reporting by parents and teachers. The BASC-2 offers rudimentary scales purporting to tap the validity of the informants' responses, but again, no validity data exist on these scales. The CBCL contains no validity scales whatsoever. Again, the clinician must use these tests with caution because they are so face valid that they are easily distorted by an informant with little knowledge of given clinical conditions.

Structured Interview Techniques

The Structured Interview of Reported Symptoms (SIRS) is the only available, well-validated, structured interview technique for identifying malingerers.[21] Only 2 studies have examined its utility among children. Rogers and his colleagues[18] tested the technique in a group of adolescents who were in a court-referred treatment program. They suggested lowering the cutoff score for identifying probable malingering from greater than or equal to 3 scales failed to greater or equal to 2 scales failed improved the power of the instrument. Dearth[22] compared a group of adolescent community volunteers instructed to malinger with a group of adolescent psychiatric patients on various tests of malingering, including the SIRS. The reported versus observed scale of the SIRS was found to be particularly useful in identifying the simulators.

Symptom Validity Testing

Symptom validity tests are psychological techniques that mimic genuine cognitive tests, but are in fact designed to assess for effort or intentional underperformance rather than actual cognitive abilities. Generally these tests use a floor-effect method of detecting malingering; individuals who score lower than the typical scores of genuinely impaired individuals are marked as suspect for malingering. Some of the more widely used of these tests include the Test of Memory Malingering (TOMM),[23] the Computerized Assessment of Response Bias (CARB),[24] Green's Word Memory Test (WMT),[25] and Green's Medical Symptom Validity Test.[26] Just as children may attempt to deceive clinicians by overreporting symptoms, so they may also malinger by acting as though they have cognitive deficits. As previously described, case reports[6,22] have identified noncredible performances in children in the context of secondary gain as well as studies using symptom validity tests in groups of children.[27] In a recent, large study of 193 children referred for evaluation after a mild traumatic brain injury, 17% of the children failed a symptom validity test within 1 year of the injury.[28]

Numerous studies have examined the performance of children on these and other common symptom validity tests. The most-researched test appears to be the TOMM, with 10 studies identified that measure the performance of children on the test. Even children as young as 5 years of age[29] typically score at or higher than the recommended cutoff scores for adults on this test (45/50). Likewise, children as young as 7 years of age taking the WMT appear to score higher than adult cutoffs, particularly if they have a third-grade or higher reading level.[29,30] On the CARB, children older than 11 years rarely fail the test.[31] The TOMM and WMT in particular, therefore, appear to be of use to the practitioner concerned about intentional underperformance in child patients.

The Validity Indicator Profile (VIP)[32] is a unique test for cognitive malingering in that it uses a strategy unlike the other tests to identify malingerers. On the VIP, the examinee is asked to respond to items requiring verbal and nonverbal reasoning that are presented in a random order, rather than in the typical easier-to-harder order of all published intelligence tests. Thus, the examinee cannot discern by placement alone the difficulty of each item. After the test is completed, a computer program scores the performance of the examinee and it is examined for unlikely patterns, such as an examinee who is successful on harder items but fails easier ones or one who performs more poorly than chance on any set of items. This test, because of its focus on reasoning ability rather than memory skills, would seem to be an excellent choice to identify children presenting with unlikely intellectual deficits. However, no research has been done on this test with children. Even so, the face-valid nature of this test means that it could be used to identify inconsistency in a child's performance, absent any formal determination of malingering.

EVALUATING THE CHILD

The previous data suggest that malingering or deception in children in the context of mental health evaluations is a common event. Clinicians should be aware of its possibility and assess children for it, particularly in the context of forensic evaluations or evaluations with a known incentive for apparent impairment (eg, ADHD evaluations for psychostimulant medications). A 2-step assessment process is suggested whereby all children are screened during the course of evaluations for malingering and children identified as suspect are then further assessed for its likelihood.

Screening During the Evaluation

The clinician should be alert to the possibility of malingering or deception in all patients, regardless of age. A routine part of each assessment should be consideration of potential motivations to underperform or to present oneself as unduly pathologic. These motivations may include financial incentives, such as the child (or his parents) who is engaged in a personal injury lawsuit or seeking disability benefits. Other potential motives may include avoidance of school or job responsibilities. Some children malinger learning disorders to obtain special accommodations in the classroom. And, as previously alluded to, children being evaluated for psychostimulant, anxiolytic, or opioid medications may have powerful motivations to present as more impaired or ill than is actually true. If any of these conditions are present, the clinician should consider the potential for malingering behavior.

Another screening tool is to evaluate the reports given by both the child and parents for consistency with one another. If the child and parent give notably differing histories or symptom reports, this is an issue for concern and further exploration. For example, a child reporting constant severely depressed mood when the parents report no overtly observed listlessness, anhedonia, or crying spells, would raise concerns.

Each child should be screened for differences between the symptom reports of the child/parent with known indices of the child's function, such as reports of activities of daily living functioning, teacher reports, report cards, review of other medical or mental health records, and with the clinician's observations of the child's functioning during the interview itself. The child who is reported to be debilitated by anxiety but who reportedly participates in a range of school activities and displays no autonomic arousal during the mental status examination, for example, would be especially suspect. A child who describes himself as suffering from severe attentional problems, but who is making good grades and displays no distractibility during the interview, would also be marked for concern.

Each child's illness presentation should also be compared with what is known about the manifestation of given psychiatric syndromes in children. As previously noted, this is an area in which the clinician usually has the advantage over patients because clinicians generally have much more experience with individuals who have the disorder that is potentially being feigned. Presumably, for example, the clinician will have worked with many psychotic patients. A child who describes vivid visual hallucinations and prominent auditory hallucinations, but who displays no distraction by internal stimuli, no alogia, no delusions, and no overall deterioration in social functioning, would of course be suspect for malingered psychosis. A child who presents with apparent amnesia for overlearned personal information (eg, name, date of birth, names of parents, names of siblings, age, and so forth) after a mild head injury would be quite suspect for malingering, as such symptoms are exceedingly rare occurrences in genuine patients.

Other specific behaviors have often been observed in malingering patients, as previously described. Many malingering patients give near-miss responses on standard mental status and information questions (eg, missing the date, month, and year by one digit; "What is 3 + 5?" "9"; "What are the colors in the American flag?" "Red, white, and green"). Presumably this occurs because when asked patients' minds produce the correct answer and it is much easier to alter the correct answer slightly than to generate a totally novel response. Assent to pseudosymptoms (eg, endorsing "The furniture in my room often changes color" or "I'm always seeing faces outside my window") should be considered. The author has found it useful with patients who assent to severe but potentially realistic symptoms of mental illness, such as prominent auditory hallucinations, to offer highly unlikely symptom combinations. For example, patients who report frequent auditory hallucinations can be asked if they are always accompanied by sudden feelings of hot or cold, or if the voices seem to come from closets and not from elsewhere. Behavior of this nature should always raise concerns for potential malingering.

Formal Assessment for Malingering

The author recommends formal, detailed assessment for deception for any child who presents with one or more of the previously mentioned behaviors or who has a known potential motivation for malingering. It may not be possible to perform a comprehensive assessment during the initial evaluation, but subsequent evaluation or referral to a forensic child psychologist should be pursued. Although the following tests and techniques are most often performed by psychologists, there is no reason that the psychiatrist with sufficient training and experience in standardized testing cannot effectively use these measures in clinical or forensic practice.

A cornerstone of comprehensive malingering assessment is the review of the child's records. Report cards, pediatrician records, teacher reports, the mental health records of other clinicians, and, in cases of alleged neurologic insult, emergency room records and neurologic examination records (eg, magnetic resonance imaging, electroencephalogram, and so forth) should always be sought and obtained if possible. This review will offer the evaluator a more detailed account of patients' apparent symptoms, as well as more information about the nature of the alleged illness. For example, a child presenting with alleged ADHD whose school records reflect little or no academic difficulties or a child with alleged severe cognitive involvement after what record review shows to have been a mild head injury, would be instances of clearly inconsistent data that would deserve an explanation.

Despite their weaknesses as measures of malingering, objective self-reported and other-reported personality testing or behavioral rating should be obtained. For children younger than 12 years of age, this would include measures such as the BASC-2 completed by the child, parents, and teacher. For teenagers, a self-report inventory, such as the MMPI-A or Adolescent Psychopathology Scale, should be completed. Although the validity scales on these instruments are untested as measures of malingering, large divergences from the norm or notable inconsistencies among informants may yield valuable information to the clinician.

Finally, symptom validity testing should be pursued with children who have known motivations for malingering or whose screening evaluations raise concerns. The TOMM, for example, has sufficiently established validity for use with even young children (ie, as young as 5 years of age). The Word Memory Test can be used with confidence with children who have at least a third-grade reading level. Although these tests are not commonly used with children, in light of the frequency of children who fail these instruments, the author thinks that they should be used much more frequently, particularly in forensic evaluations.

SUMMARY

It is apparent that children may attempt to deceive adults and are often successful at doing so. The clinical or forensic mental health evaluation setting is no exception. Children can and do misrepresent their symptoms, potentially for many motivations, including malingering. This area has been less than fully developed in the research literature, but more and more work is being done. A convergence can be discerned in the research to date, in that it has been shown that a substantial proportion of children do misrepresent their symptoms. The clinician or forensic expert has many tools at their disposal to detect this type of behavior. Data from the interview, the mental status examination, behavioral testing, and formal testing for malingering behavior can assist the clinician in identifying children who are being less than forthright in presenting their symptoms.

REFERENCES

1. Faust D, Hart K, Guilmette TJ. Pediatric malingering: the capacity of children to fake believable deficits on neuropsychological testing. J Consult Clin Psychol 1988;56(4):578–82.
2. Bigler ED. Neuropsychology and malingering: comment on Faust, Hart, and Guilmette (1988). J Consult Clin Psychol 1990;58(2):244–7.
3. Halpert E. On lying and the lie of a toddler. Psychoanal Q 2000;69(4):659–75.
4. Lewis M, Stanger C, Sullivan MW. Deception in 3-year-olds. Dev Psychol 1989;25: 439–43.
5. Talwar V, Lee K, Bala N, et al. Children's conceptual knowledge of lying and its relation to their actual behaviors: implications for court competence examinations. Law Hum Behav 2002;26(4):395–415.
6. Lu PH, Boone KB. Suspect cognitive symptoms in a 9-year-old child: malingering by proxy? Clin Neuropsychol 2002;16(1):90–6.
7. Conti RP. Malingered ADHD in adolescents diagnosed with conduct disorder: a brief note. Psychol Rep 2004;94(3 Pt 1):987–8.
8. Harrison AG, Edwards MJ, Parker KC. Identifying students faking ADHD: preliminary findings and strategies for detection. Arch Clin Neuropsychol 2007;22(5): 577–88.
9. Gunn D, Batchelor J, Jones M. Detection of simulated memory impairment in 6- to 11-year-old children. Child Neuropsychol 2010;16(2):105–18.
10. Heilbronner RL, Sweet JJ, Morgan JE, et al. American Academy of Clinical Neuropsychology Consensus Conference Statement on the neuropsychological assessment of effort, response bias, and malingering. Clin Neuropsychol 2009;23(7):1093–129.
11. Slick DJ, Sherman EM, Iverson GL. Diagnostic criteria for malingered neurocognitive dysfunction: proposed standards for clinical practice and research. Clin Neuropsychol 1999;13(4):545–61.
12. Kovacs M. Children's Depression Inventory manual. North Tonawanda (NY): Multi-Health Systems, Inc; 1992.
13. Achenbach TM. Manual for the Child Behavior Checklist. Burlington (VT): University of Vermont; 1991.
14. Briere J. Trauma Symptom Checklist for Children. Odessa (FL): Psychological Assessment Resources; 1996.
15. Reynolds CR, Kamphaus RW. Behavior Assessment System for Children manual. 2nd edition. Bloomington (MN): Pearson Assessments; 2004.
16. Kirk, Hutaff-Lee, Kirkwood MW. Utility of the self-report BASC-2 validity indicators in identifying suboptimal effort after pediatric mild TBI. The Clinical Neuropsychologist 2010;24(4):627.
17. Butcher JN, Williams CL, Graham JR, et al. MMPI-A manual for administration, scoring, and interpretation. Minneapolis (MN): University of Minnesota Press; 1992.
18. Rogers R, Hinds JD, Sewell KW. Feigning psychopathology among adolescent offenders: validation of the SIRS, MMPI-A, and SIMS. J Pers Assess 1996; 67(2):244–57.
19. Stein LA, Graham JR, Williams CL. Detecting fake-bad MMPI-A profiles. J Pers Assess 1995;65(3):415–27.
20. Reynolds WR. Adolescent psychopathology scale: administration and interpretation manual. Lutz (FL): Psychological Assessment Resources, Inc; 1998.
21. Rogers R, Bagby RM, Dickens SE. Structured Interview of Reported Symptoms (SIRS) and Professional Manual. Odessa (FL): Psychological Assessment Resources; 1992.

22. Dearth CMS. Cross-validation of malingering tests for adolescent forensic evaluations [dissertation]. Lexington (KY): University of Kentucky; 2006.
23. Tombaugh T. Test of Memory Malingering. Toronto: Multi-Health Systems, Inc; 1996.
24. Allen LM, Conder RL, Green P, et al. CARB '97: computerized assessment of response bias: manual. Durham (NC): Cognisyst; 1997.
25. Green P. Green's Word Memory Test for Microsoft Windows. Edmonton (Canada): Green's Publishing; 2003.
26. Green P. Green's Medical Symptom Validity Test (MSVT) for Microsoft Windows user's manual. Edmonton (Canada): Green's Publishing; 2003.
27. Macallister WS, Nakhutina L, Bender HA, et al. Assessing effort during neuropsychological evaluation with the TOMM in children and adolescents with epilepsy. Child Neuropsychol 2009;1–11.
28. Kirkwood MW. Testing for noncredible effort in pediatric assessment: Why, When, and How. Presented at the American Academy of Clinical Neuropsychology's 8th annual meeting. Chicago (IL), June 18, 2010.
29. Constantinou M, McCaffrey RJ. Using the TOMM for evaluating children's effort to perform optimally on neuropsychological measures. Child Neuropsychol 2003; 9(2):81–90.
30. Green P, Flaro L. Word memory test performance in children. Child Neuropsychol 2003;9(3):189–207.
31. Courtney JC, Dinkins JP, Allen LM III, et al. Age related effects in children taking the computerized assessment of response bias and word memory test. Child Neuropsychol 2003;9(2):109–16.
32. Frederick RI. Validity Indicator Profile manual. Minneapolis (MN): National Computer Systems, Inc; 1997.

Ridiculous Statements by Mental Health Experts

William Bernet, MD*

KEYWORDS

- Testimony • Expert witness • Children and adolescents
- Forensic psychiatry

The professional activities of forensic mental health practitioners are guided by the standards of practice for conducting particular types of evaluations and the ethical principles that have been published by professional organizations. For example, the American Academy of Child and Adolescent Psychiatry,[1] the American Psychiatric Association,[2] the American Academy of Psychiatry and the Law,[3] and the American Psychological Association[4] have published ethical principles for their members. These organizations have also developed guidelines or practice parameters that help define the standards of practice. For example, the American Psychological Association prepared *Specialty Guidelines for Forensic Psychology*.[5] The American Academy of Child and Adolescent Psychiatry developed a "Practice Parameter for Child and Adolescent Forensic Evaluations."[6] There are also major textbooks that give guidance to both trainees and practitioners, such as *Principles and Practice of Child and Adolescent Forensic Mental Health*,[7] *Clinical Handbook of Psychiatry and the Law*,[8] and *Principles and Practice of Forensic Psychiatry*.[9] These publications are only examples; there are many published documents that may reflect that standard of practice for mental health professionals. Of course, the standard of practice in a case is ultimately determined not by a practice guideline but by the circumstances and details of the particular case.

DISAGREEMENT AMONG EXPERTS

It is not unusual for mental health experts to disagree when they prepare dueling reports, testify at depositions and trials, and publish articles in the professional literature. It is usually a sign of constructive dialog when experts compare notes and try to understand how they came to different conclusions. For example, opposing experts may have collected incompatible or even contradictory data during the course of their

Dr Bernet has nothing to disclose.
Department of Psychiatry, Vanderbilt University School of Medicine, Nashville, TN, USA
* 1601 23rd Avenue South, Suite 3050, Nashville, TN 37212.
E-mail address: william.bernet@vanderbilt.edu

Child Adolesc Psychiatric Clin N Am 20 (2011) 557–564
doi:10.1016/j.chc.2011.03.003

respective evaluations or the experts may have collected the same data and then disagreed about the implications or conclusions that follow from the data. In many circumstances, there may simply be an honest difference of opinion because of varying interpretations of nuances that were observed in the case.

In some cases, however, disagreement among the experts occurs because an expert has employed a methodology that is far outside the usual procedure or has analyzed data in an idiosyncratic and presumably self-serving manner. After proceeding down the wrong path, the expert may arrive at conclusions that are highly implausible. On some occasions, which are unusual, testimony by a mental health expert may be so deviant from accepted ethical principles and standards of practice that it may be called ridiculous. Ridiculous, which evolved from the Latin word for ridicule, means absurd, preposterous, or silly.

There are at least 3 problems with ridiculous statements by mental health experts. First, in a trial, the trier of fact may believe the ridiculous testimony and arrive at an erroneous legal conclusion. Second, the trier of fact and other individuals involved in the case may recognize that the testimony is ridiculous, which would damage the reputation and credibility of the expert who made the statement. Third, preposterous statements or conclusions expressed by one expert may diminish the respect of judges and attorneys for the opinions of all mental health experts.

FIVE VIGNETTES

This article considers 5 situations (based on formal reports, testimony at trial, or professional writing) in which a mental health expert made ridiculous statements or arrived at ridiculous conclusions. In some of these cases the expert appeared to adopt nonstandard methods of assessment and arrived at illogical conclusions and recommendations for the purpose of favoring the side that retained them. Of course, the role of an expert as a hired gun may compromise the reputation of legitimate, ethical experts. These cases, which are disguised, occurred in several different states and settings. The actual names of the mental health experts and evaluees are not used. Each vignette is followed by a brief discussion. Following the case illustrations, the author provides several suggestions to aid mental health practitioners in avoiding this type of error.

Pellet Gun and Neuropsychology

Andy, a 10-year-old boy, was playing at a friend's house. The friend had recently received a gift of an air rifle and was trying to figure out how to pump up the air rifle for maximum velocity. The air rifle did not shoot BBs, but small pellets. Andy's friend accidentally fired the pellet gun and hit Andy in the left side of his forehead. Although initially it seemed that Andy had sustained only a superficial injury, later in the day he became unusually somnolent. At a local emergency room, a brain scan revealed that the pellet was lodged in the left temporal region of his brain. Andy was treated to reduce the elevated pressure around his brain and his most obvious symptoms resolved. The neurosurgeons decided to not remove the pellet.

Andy's parents initiated a legal action against the manufacturer of the pellet gun, and he was evaluated by forensic neuropsychologists for both the plaintiffs (Andy's parents) and the defendant (the gun manufacturer) of the lawsuit. The forensic neuropsychologists were not asked to address the liability of the gun manufacturer, but they attempted to determine if Andy had been permanently damaged by this head injury. For example, they tried to compare Andy's cognitive and emotional functioning before and after the injury. The forensic neuropsychologist, Dr A, who was hired by the defendant, the gun manufacturer, made an unusual, ridiculous statement in his report: "I am not aware of any scientific basis for saying that this type of injury causes permanent brain damage."

Discussion

On the face of it, the statement by Dr A was highly implausible. It seemed extremely unlikely that the average neurosurgeon, psychologist, psychiatrist, or parent would consider a penetrating injury to a child's temporal lobe to be a benign event. Actually, it was easy to show that there were articles in the medical literature regarding the consequences of this type of head injury in children.[10-13] Ultimately, the legal team for the defendant did not use Dr A at trial because his opinion was unbelievable.

Damages from Street Hockey

A school counselor, Mr Bunson, sexually molested about 10 students, all boys, at a public middle school. After the sexual abuse was disclosed and investigated, Mr Bunson was arrested, tried, convicted, and imprisoned. The parents of several of the students initiated a lawsuit against school personnel and the board of education. Both the plaintiffs (the parents) and the defendants (the school personnel and the board of education) hired forensic mental health experts. Those mental health experts were not asked to address the liability of the defendants, but to assess whether the children had been psychologically damaged by the sexual abuse. Also, the mental health experts were asked to estimate the current and future treatment, if any, these children will require to recover from the sexual abuse.

Obviously, Mr Bunson had seriously molested some of the boys who had been injured by the abuse that they experienced. However, one of the alleged victims, Bradley, alleged that Mr Bunson had touched him in an extremely brief, superficial manner. Specifically, Bradley related that he and several other students were playing street hockey with Mr Bunson during an after-school program. During that play activity, the front part of Mr Bunson's body bumped into the back part of Bradley's body. Bradley turned to Mr Bunson and said, "Get away from me! I'm not gay!" The mental health expert for the plaintiffs, Dr B, thought that Bradley had been psychologically injured by that experience and she gave him the diagnosis of posttraumatic stress disorder.

Dr B recommended the same treatment regimen for Bradley, who had a minimal unpleasant experience with Mr Bunson, as she did for the boys who had been significantly abused. Dr B, the expert for the plaintiffs, recommended a multimodal treatment program for Bradley, which consisted of the following components: weekly individual therapy for 10 years; weekly group counseling for 3 years; weekly family therapy for 3 years; weekly private tutoring for 6 years; as well as sports activities, crisis intervention, health monitoring, and vocational testing. The expert estimated that Bradley would need 1500 hours of counseling and other interventions to recover from his brief encounter with Mr Bunson.

Discussion

It could be argued that Bradley may have been injured in some limited manner because of his relationship with Mr Bunson. However, it was ridiculous to claim that Bradley had been severely injured by a transitory event during a sports activity that lasted approximately 1 second. Also, it was ridiculous to assert that this boy might need 10 years of individual psychotherapy to recover from that experience. Dr B's absurd opinions regarding Bradley's need for future treatment may have diminished the weight of her opinions regarding the other victims of Mr Bunson.

A Child who was not Abused

The mother of a 3-year-old boy, Charlie, repeatedly took him to primary care physicians, emergency room personnel, and pediatric urologists because she thought her son had been sexually abused by his father. The parents were divorced and the mother sought to exclude the father from the child's life.

Ultimately, the child protection service (CPS) became involved and a CPS worker interviewed Charlie in his bedroom at his mother's home. In that interview, Charlie's statements were confused, irrelevant, and incomprehensible. Charlie did not provide any meaningful or intelligible information. He apparently was not capable of giving a simple, coherent description of a past event. When asked suggestive questions, Charlie tried to give answers that he thought would please the interviewer. When pushed to answer questions beyond his scope of knowledge, Charlie gave nonsensical and fantastical answers, such as saying his father hammered his penis with a shovel. Although there was zero forensically useful content in that interview, CPS staff concluded that Charlie's father sexually abused the boy.

At a subsequent child custody trial, a forensic psychologist hired by the mother, Dr C, testified that the allegations based on the CPS interview were more credible than the forensic evaluation conducted several months later. Dr C testified that the chaotic, disorganized CPS interview indicated that Charlie had been sexually abused by his father because, "I've interviewed hundreds of children, where sexual abuse allegations have been made, and when you get a situation like this the reporting of the child contemporaneous with the allegations is significantly and profoundly more real than what the child would report 6 months or a year later." In the end, the trial judge disregarded the testimony by Dr C and the court of appeals upheld the decision of the judge.

Discussion

In this case, Dr C was basing his opinion on an abstract, general principle: earlier interviews are more reliable than later interviews. The expert had the idea that the general principle was more important than the actual data collected during the investigation. Dr C's testimony was preposterous because he had never listened to the recording or read the transcript of the CPS interview. He had expressed a strong opinion about the ultimate question of the hearing without ever interviewing the child or reviewing the actual data of the CPS interview. Dr C's methodology violated ethical standard 9.01b of the American Psychological Association: "Except as noted in 9.01c, psychologists provide opinions of the psychological characteristics of individuals only after they have conducted an examination adequate to support their statements or conclusions."[4]

Interviewing a Nonverbal Child

When David was 6 years old he attended a special education preschool program at a public elementary school. David had severe mental retardation and a developmental psychologist said he exhibited "a severe receptive and expressive language disorder." Sadly, David and other students in his special education class were mistreated by their teacher, Ms Downing. According to witnesses, Ms Downing restrained David on his cot during naptime because otherwise he would get up and walk around. Ms Downing reportedly hit David with a yardstick and took him outside the building in the winter without his coat on. When the abuse became known, David's parents sued the school system for allowing the teacher to abuse David.

The family's mental health expert, Dr D, evaluated David, which included an interview that was electronically recorded. In the interview, David made various sounds but no words. He was looking at a book and did not respond when Dr D asked him to point to a boy and a person and look at a tree and a bird. David did not appear to understand what Dr D said to him. Dr D repeatedly tried to communicate with David. He repeatedly asked David what he remembered about his teacher, Ms Downing. He repeatedly asked questions, such as "What did Ms Downing do to you?" At no time did David give a meaningful response, either verbal or nonverbal, to Dr D's questions.

David was also interviewed by the mental health expert hired by the school system. In that interview, David was nonverbal. He was able to imitate the examiner and clap his hands. At times he played a simple game of handing objects back and forth. He tried to put items of interest in his mouth. David was able to use a colored marker to make random marks on paper but was not able to make a scribble. He was not able to stack one block on top of another.

Dr D's written report was notable because he claimed to derive significant meaning from David's activities during the forensic interview. Dr D stated, "I was impressed that my introducing the topic of Ms Downing produces marked behavioral change that appears very meaningful. He was remarkably negatively reactive to discussion of Ms Downing. Introduction of her name leads to David's agitation and oppositional behavior." In fact, however, the electronic recording of the interview revealed no reaction at all to Dr D's questions regarding Ms Downing.

Discussion
In this case, the plaintiff's expert, Dr D, totally misrepresented David's activities and reactions that occurred during his forensic interview, to the point of being ridiculous. Fortunately, the interview was electronically recorded so it could be examined by the expert for the defendant and other individuals involved in the case. A careful review of the digital file revealed that David did not appear to understand anything Dr D said and did not respond to Dr D's questions in any meaningful manner.

Diagnostic and Statistical Manual of Mental Disorders (Fifth Edition) Controversy

Since 2008, the author of this article and his colleagues have campaigned that the concept of parental alienation become a new diagnosis to be included in the Diagnostic and Statistical Manual of Mental Disorders, Fifth Edition (DSM-5). They submitted a formal proposal to the DSM-5 Task Force in 2009 and published their proposal in a journal article[14] and a book[15] in 2010. The authors' definition of parental alienation was a mental condition in which "a child—usually one whose parents are engaged in a high-conflict divorce—allies himself or herself strongly with one parent (the preferred parent) and rejects a relationship with the other parent (the alienated parent) without legitimate justification."[15]

The proposal that parental alienation become a DSM-5 diagnosis generated a good deal of discussion among mental health professionals. Many psychiatrists and psychologists agreed that parental alienation should be considered a relational problem, but not a mental disorder in DSM-5. Some of the discussion regarding that proposal, especially comments on Web sites and Internet blogs, was extremely negative and hostile to the concept of parental alienation. One of the opponents of the author's proposal regarding parental alienation was Dr E, a well-known psychiatrist. Dr E published his opinions in a mental health newspaper, which were extremely critical of both the concept of parental alienation and the advocates of the proposal, perhaps to the point of being libelous. In his essay, Dr E referred to parental alienation syndrome (PAS) as "this bit of junk science invented by a psychiatrist...." In referring to the proposal that parental alienation become a diagnosis in DSM-5, Dr E said, "In recent years, the ball has been picked up by 'father's rights' groups who don't like to be interfered with when they are sexually abusing their children. This group has petitioned the DSM task force to include PAS in the publication."

Dr E clearly stated that individuals who proposed that parental alienation should become a diagnosis in DSM-5 engaged in child sexual abuse. In response to Dr E's ridiculous statements, at least 8 mental health and legal professionals wrote letters to the editor of the mental health newspaper that published Dr E's essay. Dr E was required to correct his outrageous statements and make amends. In a subsequent issue he said, "I apologize for suggesting that all fathers who accuse mothers of PAS are sexually abusing their children. That was clearly an overstatement that I retract." Also, "I do not deny that parental alienation occurs and that a lot of people are hurt when there is an alienator."

Discussion

In this example, Dr E's ridiculous statement did not occur directly in a legal context, such as an expert report or testimony. However, the proposal that parental alienation be included in DSM-5 has both clinical and legal implications and Dr E was clearly expressing opinions as an expert on that topic. In the previous examples of ridiculous statements in this article, the give and take between various opinions played out in the form of opposing expert reports or experts battling in a courtroom. In this example involving a controversial proposal that is being considered by DSM-5 personnel, the dialog took place in a public forum.

SUGGESTIONS FOR FORENSIC PRACTITIONERS

It may be extremely frustrating when a forensic expert is confronted with a ridiculous statement or opinion in a legal setting or other public venue. The expert may feel totally unprepared to analyze or discuss an assertion that seems to be preposterous and have no foundation. Here are suggestions that forensic experts may consider if they find themselves in that situation.

When testifying, do not be reluctant to say another expert is flatly wrong if you know that is the case, even if you do not have published research on hand to back up your statement. For example, in the case of alleged sexual molestation while playing street hockey, it would seem preposterous to most jurors for the plaintiffs' expert to say that the child needed 10 years of individual psychotherapy to recover from being bumped during a game. It is a truism that minor problems should require only minimal psychotherapy.

If you know ahead of time that another expert is going to make a ridiculous statement, do some research and secure references that support your position. For example, regarding the case in which a child was shot in the head with a pellet from an air rifle, the typical mental health expert would probably not be familiar with research pertaining to that type of injury. It was easy, however, to find review articles by neurologists and neurosurgeons regarding that topic.

If you feel that a mental health expert violated the ethical precepts of their own profession in making a ridiculous statement, consider filing a complaint with the relevant committee or board of ethics. For example, the psychologist who testified about the importance of a particular interview without reviewing either the audiotape or the transcript of the interview appeared to violate one of the ethical standards of the American Psychological Association. In such a case, it would be appropriate to refer the matter to the Ethics Committee of the American Psychological Association for their consideration.

However, if the expert's ridiculous statement occurred in a public forum, it might be possible to redress the situation in the same manner. If the statement occurred in a publication, contact the editor promptly. If the statement occurred on television, contact the producer of the show. It may be helpful to let colleagues know what has occurred, because they may also want to contact the editor or producer of the offensive statement. Typically, you should insist that the statement be retracted or corrected.

Preventing an error is almost always preferable to correcting the error. Mental health professionals who intend to offer an expert opinion should limit their comments to topics that they thoroughly understand. Otherwise, they may accidentally arrive at a ridiculous conclusion and embarrass themselves when testifying. Also, forensic practitioners should make a regular practice of asking a colleague to review the draft of a report before it is finalized. Ask the colleague to read the report with a critical eye and question your assumptions and conclusions. A person reading the final draft of your report for the first time may be able to point out small errors as well as major gaffes in your text.

SUMMARY

Mental health experts need to improve their image and reputation as credible witnesses. There is no way to avoid an occasional battle of the experts, and most people understand that honest and experienced experts may arrive at different conclusions. However, statements that are ridiculous or preposterous are damaging in several ways: to the reputation of the expert making the ridiculous statement; by extension, to the credibility of other experts; and perhaps to the outcome of the case, if the ridiculous statement is believed by the trier of fact. To minimize the frequency of that sad occurrence, mental health experts should scrutinize their own reports and testimony as well as the work of their colleagues.

REFERENCES

1. American Academy of Child and Adolescent Psychiatry. Code of Ethics. Washington, DC: American Academy of Child and Adolescent Psychiatry; 2009.
2. American Psychiatric Association. The principles of medical ethics with annotations especially applicable to psychiatry. Arlington (VA): American Psychiatric Association; 2009.
3. American Academy of Psychiatry and the Law. Ethics guidelines for the practice of forensic psychiatry. Bloomfield (CT): American Academy of Psychiatry and the Law; 2005.
4. American Psychological Association. Ethical principles of psychologists and code of conduct. Am Psychol 2002;57:1060–73.
5. American Psychological Association. Specialty guidelines for forensic psychology. Washington, DC: American Psychological Association; 2010.
6. American Academy of Child and Adolescent Psychiatry. Practice parameter for child and adolescent forensic evaluations. J Am Acad Child Adolesc Psychiatry, in press.
7. Benedek E, Ash P, Scott CL. Principles and practice of child and adolescent forensic mental health. 2nd edition. Washington, DC: American Psychiatric Publishing, Inc; 2010.
8. Appelbaum PS, Gutheil TG. Clinical handbook of psychiatry and the law. 4th edition. Philadelphia: Lippincott, Williams, Wilkins; 2007.
9. Rosner R. Principles and practice of forensic psychiatry. 2nd edition. London: Arnold; 2003.

10. Miner CE, Cabrera JA, Ford E, et al. Intracranial penetration due to BB air rifle injuries. Neurosurgery 1986;19:952–4.
11. Jamjoom AB, Rawlinson JN, Clarke PM. Air gun injuries of the brain. Injury 1989; 20:344–6.
12. Bond SJ, Schnier GC, Miller FB. Air-powered guns: too much firepower to be a toy. J Trauma 1996;41:674–8.
13. Demuren OA, Mehta DS. Spontaneous gun pellet migration in the brain. West Afr J Med 1997;16:117–20.
14. Bernet W, Boch-Galhau WV, Baker AJ, et al. Parental alienation, DSM-V, and ICD-11. Am J Fam Ther 2010;38:176–87.
15. Bernet W. Parental alienation, DSM-5, and ICD-11. Springfield (IL): Charles C Thomas; 2010.

The Child and Adolescent Track in the Forensic Fellowship

Charles Scott, MD

KEYWORDS

- Child and adolescent forensic psychiatry
- Forensic psychiatry residency
- Child and adolescent forensic psychiatrist
- ACGME forensic psychiatry program requirements

The term child forensic psychiatrist generally refers to psychiatrists who have completed residency training in 3 areas accredited by the American Council on Graduate Medical Education (ACGME): general psychiatry (ie, adult psychiatry), child and adolescent psychiatry, and forensic psychiatry. As a forensic psychiatry residency training director, who is trained and certified in these areas, I have been impressed by the increasing number of child and adolescent psychiatrists who are now seeking a forensic psychiatry residency program that specifically offers a child forensic track. Reasons commonly cited by child and adolescent–trained psychiatrists pursuing a forensic psychiatry residency include the following:

1. A desire to assist underserved youth who have interfaced with the juvenile justice system
2. A specific interest in forensic psychiatry to include forensic assessments of both adults and juveniles
3. A need to better understand issues related to evaluating allegations of abuse, particularly sexual abuse allegations
4. An interest in having a broad-based practice with a combination of private forensic work and clinical duties
5. A desire to obtain public policy expertise relevant to child and adolescent psychiatric issues
6. An interest in testifying in court based on prior experiences in their general and/or child and adolescent psychiatry training.

The author has nothing to disclose.
Division of Psychiatry and the Law, Department of Psychiatry & Behavioral Sciences, University of California, Davis Medical Center, 2230 Stockton Boulevard, 2nd Floor, Sacramento, CA 95817, USA
E-mail address: charles.scott@ucdmc.ucdavis.edu

Child Adolesc Psychiatric Clin N Am 20 (2011) 565–575
doi:10.1016/j.chc.2011.03.010
1056-4993/11/$ – see front matter © 2011 Elsevier Inc. All rights reserved.

childpsych.theclinics.com

Many child and adolescent psychiatrist applicants seeking a child-focused track cite a combination of the reasons listed earlier, whereas others acknowledge that they have a general curiosity regarding child and adolescent forensic psychiatry without a clear understanding of why they feel compelled to extend their lengthy training for an additional year.

This article refers to a child and adolescent psychiatry track within a forensic residency program as a child forensic track, and provides practical guidance for forensic psychiatry residency directors on how to implement a child forensic track within the existing ACGME Program Requirements for Graduate Medical Education in Forensic Psychiatry. Important aspects to understand when designing a child and adolescent–focused track include an understanding of ACGME program requirements for residency training in general psychiatry and child and adolescent psychiatry, qualifications of forensic psychiatry faculty to teach child and adolescent forensic psychiatry, child-focused learning sites appropriate for forensic psychiatry residency experiences, a review of how core ACGME program requirements typically applied to adult forensic cases may also be met through child and adolescent equivalent didactic and clinical experiences, and suggestions for scholarly activities for the child and adolescent psychiatrist enrolled in the forensic psychiatry residency.

FORENSIC REQUIREMENTS OF ACGME

When reviewing the ACGME program requirements for both general psychiatry and child and adolescent psychiatry residency programs, it is clear that forensic issues are only minimally represented. Such limited exposure to forensic issues further supports the need for a child forensic track for child and adolescent psychiatrists seeking additional training in child and adolescent forensic psychiatry. There are only 3 mentions of forensic psychiatry experiences or exposure noted in the program requirements for general psychiatry:

1. During the second through the fourth years, the didactic curriculum should include "the legal aspects of psychiatric practice"[1]
2. The psychiatric curriculum must "provide residents with direct experience in progressive responsibility for patient management."[1] The 2 references to forensic psychiatry relevant to this specific guideline include the following:
   a. The general psychiatry resident is required to have exposure to emergency room assessments that must include "knowledge of relevant issues in forensic psychiatry"[1]
   b. A forensic psychiatry experience qualifying as part of a psychiatric curriculum is defined as an "experience under the supervision of a psychiatrist in evaluation of patients with forensic problems."[1]

The program requirements for child and adolescent psychiatry are similarly sparse in regards to mandatory forensic training, with the only references to forensic experiences for the child and adolescent resident noted as follows:

1. Residents must have an organized clinical "experience in legal issues relevant to child and adolescent psychiatry, which may include forensic consultation, court testimony and/or interaction with a juvenile justice system"[2]
2. The curriculum must include adequate and systematic instruction in the "recognition and management of domestic and community violence (including physical and sexual abuse, as well as neglect) as it affects children and adolescents."[2]

The forensic program requirements for both general and child and adolescent psychiatry residency programs are highlighted earlier to assist program directors in understanding the narrow forensic foundation of most trainees who are interested in pursuing a child forensic track. Therefore, a child forensic track must provide important basic forensic core competencies that should not be assumed to have been taught during either prior residency training program.

FORENSIC PSYCHIATRY TEACHING FACULTY

The ACGME program requirements require that the teaching physician faculty include at least 1 certified child and adolescent psychiatrist.[3] In addition, these guidelines emphasize that all physician faculty members (to include the child and adolescent–certified faculty member) must be certified by the American Board of Psychiatry and Neurology (ABPN) in the subspecialty of forensic psychiatry, or possess qualifications judged to be acceptable by the Residency Review Committee (RRC).[3] When considering these 2 statements together, the program requirements clearly emphasize a preference for the child and adolescent psychiatrist on the forensic faculty to be certified by the ABPN in both child and adolescent psychiatry and forensic psychiatry. Although board certification in child and adolescent psychiatry does not seem negotiable according to these guidelines, additional board certification in forensic psychiatry can be considered on a case-by-case basis if appropriate forensic qualifications are deemed acceptable by the RRC.

For forensic psychiatry residency training programs whose child and adolescent psychiatrist faculty member is not ABPN certified in forensic psychiatry, qualifications that may be forwarded to the RRC to consider as appropriate include the following:

1. Direct clinical experience in child and adolescent forensic psychiatry through provision of consultation, assessment, and/or treatment at facilities that focus on juvenile offenders. Such settings could include 1 or more of the following: juvenile detention facilities; partial day hospitalization programs, outpatient programs, or group homes for juvenile offenders; juvenile sex offender assessment and treatment programs; and/or consultation with continuation schools for juvenile delinquents
2. A developed forensic expertise in an area or areas of child and adolescent forensic psychiatry. Common areas in which child and adolescent psychiatrists may have developed expertise in the forensic arena without having completed a forensic psychiatry residency include child custody evaluations; evaluations for juvenile court (such as competency to stand trial and/or risk assessments); violence risk assessment for requesting agencies (such as schools); evaluations of abuse allegations; evaluations of psychic harm or trauma; and/or a specialized expertise in evaluations regarding standard of care
3. A developed consultation-liaison expertise that focuses on forensic issues facing child and adolescent psychiatrists in a variety of settings. Important forensic issues that may arise in the child and adolescent consultative setting and that could be considered for an acceptable qualification include legal issues related to the right to treatment, the right to refuse treatment, mandatory child abuse referrals, informed consent issues related to medications and medical procedures, involuntary commitment, and/or suicide and violence risk assessments of youth
4. A documented learning program in areas of forensic psychiatry. Such concentrated areas of learning might include a completed forensic psychiatry residency program (but not certified by ABPN), extensive forensic course work through national review

courses such as those offered by the American Academy of Psychiatry and the Law (AAPL), or attendance at relevant law school classes or a completed law school education.

Although the completion of a forensic psychiatry residency provides a critical foundation important in understanding the interface of child and adolescent psychiatry with forensic psychiatry, there are many well-regarded experts in child and adolescent forensic psychiatry who have gained their expertise through years of practical forensic experience rather than a formal forensic psychiatry residency. Therefore, the lack of certification in forensic psychiatry does not represent an absolute bar to an ABPN-certified child and adolescent psychiatrist serving on an ACGME-accredited forensic psychiatry residency faculty.

CHILD-FOCUSED LEARNING SITES

The ACGME program requirements for forensic psychiatry residency training require the program to include training experiences in 3 venues. When designing a child-focused track within the forensic residency program, the training director should consider those juvenile settings that most closely parallel the venues required by the program guidelines. The exact language for the 3 required learning venues is provided later, with suggestions for child-focused experiences that parallel the more general forensic psychiatry residency program requirements. The 3 required venues specified by ACGME for a forensic psychiatry residency program include the following:

- "Facilities in which forensic psychiatric evaluations are performed on subjects with a broad variety of psychiatric disorders, where residents can learn evaluation techniques. These may include court clinics, inpatient forensic units, outpatient forensic clinics, and private practices."[3] Child-focused facilities that match this learning venue include juvenile court clinics, juvenile detention facilities, outpatient clinics for juvenile offenders, and private practice clinics of child and adolescent forensic psychiatrists
- "Facilities that provide general psychiatric services to patients with a broad variety of psychiatric disorders, where residents can learn consultation regarding legal issues in psychiatric practice. These may include inpatient and outpatient facilities or may be specialized facilities that provide psychiatric care to correctional populations."[3] Potential parallel child-focused experiences in this arena might include child and/or adolescent psychiatry inpatient units, general hospital inpatient units, partial or day treatment programs, group homes for delinquent youth, child abuse evaluation assessment centers, and/or continuation schools that work with juveniles involved in the juvenile justice system
- "Facilities that treat persons in the correctional system, where residents can learn about the specialized treatment issues raised by these populations and settings. These facilities may include prisons, jails, hospital-based correctional units, halfway facilities, rehabilitation programs, community probation programs, forensic clinics, juvenile detention facilities, and maximum security forensic hospital facilities."[3] Examples of appropriate child forensic-focused experiences in this required category include juvenile detention facilities, facilities for juveniles whose disposition involves commitment to a correctional facility, juvenile substance abuse diversion treatment programs, juvenile probation and community monitoring programs, and juveniles who may be housed in a forensic psychiatric hospital.

Important factors to consider when organizing a child-focused clinical site are highlighted in **Box 1**.

SPECIALTY CURRICULUM FOR A CHILD-FOCUSED TRACK

According to the program requirements for forensic psychiatry residency training, "The program must possess a well-organized and effective curriculum, both didactic and clinical. The curriculum must also provide residents with direct experience in progressive responsibility for patient management."[3] The program curriculum is divided into 2 main categories: didactic curriculum and forensic experiences. The application of child-focused training experiences in each of these categories is summarized later.

Didactic Curriculum

The program requirements provide a clear mandate that the didactic curriculum must include specific didactic training in 10 areas of forensic psychiatry. Although none of these 10 areas specifically address children or adolescents, each area has a child and adolescent parallel component that is important to address in a child forensic track. **Table 1** outlines specific forensic topics noted in the 10 required didactic areas with corresponding child and adolescent forensic issues. **Table 1** is not intended to represent a comprehensive list of all subject areas for the corresponding child-focused topic but instead provides a starting point to consider when designing a child-focused didactic curriculum.

In addition to the mandated didactic curriculum outlined in **Table 1**, the program requires a law curriculum that covers issues in 3 main areas: the legal system, civil law, and criminal law. The law curriculum suggests, rather than mandates, a total of 32 topic areas that an appropriate law curriculum might encompass. Seven of the recommended 32 topic areas are specific to child and adolescent psychiatry. The child-focused track should consider making these topic areas mandatory for child and adolescent psychiatrists in the forensic psychiatry residency. Content material to consider in each of these 7 legal subject areas includes the following:

1. Children's rights:
   a. Mature minor doctrine
   b. Emancipated minor doctrine
   c. Right to confidential psychiatric treatment
   d. Right to contraception and/or abortion
   e. Right to treatment without parent's knowledge
   f. Right to refuse treatment

Box 1
Factors to consider when organizing a child forensic-focused experience

- The qualifications of the on-site supervisor, who ideally should be a certified child and adolescent psychiatrist

- The breadth of exposure the opportunity affords

- The feasibility of the site in relationship to other required aspects of the program

- The safety of the environment

- Adequate support personnel on site

Table 1
Child and adolescent forensic psychiatry curriculum

Mandatory ACGME Curriculum Topic	Corresponding Child and Adolescent Forensic Psychiatry Topic
History of forensic psychiatry	Evaluation of children's legal culpability under Roman and English common law
	US Houses of Refuge
	Creation of Juvenile Courts in the late 1800s
	Juvenile Justice and Delinquency Prevention Act
Roles and responsibilities of forensic psychiatrists	Understanding the contrasting roles in clinical vs forensic examination
	Gathering data from family, school, and other collateral resources especially relevant to juveniles
	Learning the legal responsibility for child abuse allegations that may surface during a forensic examination
Assessment of competency to stand trial	Understanding those issues unique to juvenile competency to include developmental immaturity as a potential predicate for a finding of trial incompetency
	Awareness of structured assessment instruments specific to juvenile trial competency
	Knowledge of relationship of competency evaluations to judicial waivers
Assessment of criminal responsibility	Appreciation of developmental issues to criminal intent and mens rea
	Understanding developmental issues relevant to insanity statute components
Assessment of amnesia	Understanding of childhood amnesia from birth to age 3 years
	Evaluation of claimed dissociation in regards to child abuse trauma
	Knowledge of specific techniques to evaluate amnesia claims in juveniles
Testamentary capacity	Application of testamentary capacity to an emancipated minor
Civil competency	Evaluation of an emancipated minor's ability to enter into a civil contract
	Understanding of both an emancipated minor and mature minor's ability to make medical decisions
	Competency of a minor to refuse or accept treatment
Assessment of dangerousness	Factors specific to juvenile's risk of future violence
	Knowledge regarding actuarial and structured clinical judgment in regards to juvenile risk assessment
	Understanding assessment of juvenile psychopathy and associated controversy

Assessment of the accused sexual offender	Knowledge of factors specific to juvenile sexual offending Familiarity with various sex offender risk assessment instruments Understanding of best practice treatment recommendations for juvenile sex offending
Evaluation and treatment of incarcerated individuals	Knowledge regarding the epidemiology of mental disorders among detained youth Understanding of common mental health screening and assessment instruments for incarcerated youth Appreciation of best practices treatment approaches for incarcerated youth
Ethical, administrative, and legal issues in forensic psychiatry	Appreciation of importance of knowing agency policy and procedures governing juvenile evaluations and treatment Knowledge of relevant ethical guidelines for psychiatric care and forensic evaluations of juveniles to include the American Psychiatric Association, American Academy of Child and Adolescent Psychiatry, and American Academy of Psychiatry and the Law ethical guidelines Concerns regarding child abuse, informed consent, and identification of guardian Landmark cases that deal specifically with juvenile and family issues
Legal regulation of psychiatric practice	Standards of care regarding the treatment of minors to include off-label prescribing and suicide risk assessments
Writing of a forensic report	Documentation regarding family and school sources of information Application of relevant statutory and case law to writing a forensic opinion Discussion of developmental issues relevant to legal issues of the case Identification of potential protective factors and resiliency in youth
Eyewitness testimony	Knowledge regarding memory recall and errors in children aged 3–18 years Interview effects on child witness testimony

g. Right to freedom from sexual harassment in both a school and working environment.
2. Family law:
   a. Dependency petitions
   b. Adoption issues and children
   c. Guardian *ad litem* appointments
   d. Children in Need of Services (CHINS)
   e. Families in Need of Services (FINS).
3. Structure and function of juvenile systems:
   a. History and development of juvenile court
   b. Juvenile court process with terminology used in the juvenile court process
   c. Role of the juvenile probation officer and disposition hearing
   d. Laws related to separation of youth from adults in detainment facilities.
4. Child custody determinations
   a. The doctrine of the best interests of the child
   b. National and international laws related to uniform recognition of child custody decisions and parental kidnapping.
5. Parental competence and termination of parental rights
   a. Standard of proof required for termination of parental rights
   b. Legal issues related to evaluating parental competence.
6. Child abuse and neglect
   a. Mandatory child abuse reporting statutes.
7. Developmental disability law
   a. Laws governing a free and appropriate public education and the least restrictive educational environment
   b. Legal requirements for individualized education plans.

FORENSIC EXPERIENCES

In addition to the didactic curriculum outlined earlier, the program requirements mandate that "forensic experiences must provide residents with sufficient opportunity for the psychiatric evaluation of individuals" in the following 5 areas: criminal behavior, criminal responsibility and competency to stand trial, sexual misconduct, dangerousness, and civil law and regulation of psychiatry issues.[3] There are 2 basic approaches a forensic psychiatry residency program can take to meet this requirement, either alone or in combination.

Pairing Resident with Faculty

First, each of these 5 forensic experiences can be created by pairing the forensic psychiatry resident with a child and adolescent psychiatrist who is conducting the evaluation. In this situation, the faculty member should clarify with the referral party whether there are objections from any party to the resident's observing the forensic evaluation. Because most child and adolescent psychiatric residents in the forensic program have not yet received ABPN certification or have limited forensic experience in the civil forensic psychiatry arena, attorneys are less likely to retain a forensic resident as the sole forensic expert in civil cases. Therefore, organizing a conjoint interview or observation role for the resident provides the resident with the experience of evaluating a youth who has made a psychiatric claim in the civil litigation arena. Despite potential reluctance of attorneys to privately retain a forensic psychiatry resident in civil cases, these agreements are much more feasible in evaluations of juveniles involved in the juvenile justice system.

Residents as Court-appointed Evaluators

Second, the forensic psychiatry residency programs should work with their local juvenile justice court system to approve appointment of those forensic residents, trained in child and adolescent psychiatry, to panels of experts who are court appointed to conduct forensic psychiatric evaluations of juveniles. Providing education regarding the background and training of the forensic resident to juvenile court judges, defense attorneys, and prosecutors, can both inform and reassure the court of the qualifications of the forensic resident and increase the likelihood of receiving referrals.

In addition to forensic experiences in psychiatric evaluations, the program guidelines also require that the resident have experience in the review of written records, in the preparation of a written report and/or testimony in a diversity of cases, a supervised experience in testifying in court or in mock trial simulations, and supervised training in the relevance of legal documents. All of these requirements can be met through implementing 1 or more of the following teaching strategies.

Strategy 1: Mock Trial

When working with forensic residents who are conducting psychiatric evaluations for a forensic referral, supervising child and adolescent psychiatrists should ensure that that have reviewed the relevant legal and clinical documents in the preparation of their written reports. Even if testimony is not required, conducting a mock trial experience can assist the resident in developing court testimony skills. Mock trial experiences can be divided into discrete learning modules that involve videotaped training on the presentation of appropriate credentials, challenge of credentials, presentation of direct testimony, as well as cross-examination.

Strategy 2: Library of Forensic Cases

The forensic residency program should consider developing a teaching library of forensic cases with redacted identifying information. For example, the child and adolescent psychiatric faculty member could retain a variety of forensic cases that involved a written report to the court. After redacting any identifying information, the resident is provided the written psychiatric evaluation with the identified referral question. With this initial information, the resident is assigned the following learning tasks with corresponding supervision and guidance:

- Prepare a written list of collateral records or interviews that may be important in the evaluation of this case
- Prepare a written summary of records based on additional records provided (eg, police reports, hospital records)
- Write a written forensic opinion based on the information provided. The writing of this parallel report allows a close comparison with the opinion and supportive reasoning of the supervising faculty
- Undergo a mock cross-examination by the supervising faculty member based on the summary of records and written opinion created by the resident.

Strategy 3: Affiliated Attorneys

Create a mock trial experience with an affiliated faculty attorney who provides the direct and cross-examination. Important components of creating a mock trial experience for the resident include the following:

- Provide the examining attorney with the forensic report with sufficient time in advance to prepare the examination

- Require supervising faculty to observe the mock trial and provide both verbal and written feedback
- Videotape the mock trial experience with feedback provided to the resident on areas of improvement and subsequent reexamination to assist in improved testimony skills.

Experience in Two Settings

The final 2 categories of required forensic experiences noted in the ACGME program guidelines involve the provision of care to individuals in 2 settings. The first mandate involves a consultative experience with clinicians regarding legal issues that arise in psychiatric practice. To meet this program requirement and provide a child-focused experience, the forensic residency program should develop a consultative relationship with 1 or more of the following settings: emergency rooms that service pediatric patients, hospital pediatric inpatient units or outpatient clinics, juvenile detention facilities, and/or school mental health programs. Suggested forensic pediatric consultative experiences would typically include civil commitment and dangerousness, confidentiality, decision-making competence, guardianship, and refusal of treatment.

The second required clinical experience involves the evaluation and management of acutely and chronically ill patients in correctional system such as prisons, jails, community programs, and secure facilities. The ACGME program guidelines specifically note that the residents must have at least 6 months' experience in the management of patients in correctional settings. However, no further clarification is provided regarding what this experience must encompass. A child-focused track could meet this requirement through the provision of clinical services to youth housed in juvenile detention facilities or enrolled in probation programs, adolescents incarcerated in adult facilities, and juveniles involved in youth correctional settings or secure forensic facilities.

Those forensic psychiatry residency programs that provide clinical assessments and treatment to individuals 13 years old or younger should be familiar with the program guideline that states, "Direct clinical work with children under the age of 14 years should be limited to residents who have previously completed ACGME-approved training in child and adolescent psychiatry or to residents who are under the supervision of a board certified child and adolescent psychiatrist or an individual who possesses qualifications to be acceptable by the RRC."[3]

RESIDENT SCHOLARLY ACTIVITY

A scholarly activity is the final learning activity mandated by the ACGME program requirements. In particular, the program requirements specify that "each program must provide an opportunity for residents to participate in research or other scholarly activities, and residents must participate actively in such scholarly activities."[3] Opportunities for a child and adolescent psychiatrist to meet this requirement might include 1 or more of the following experiences:

1. Conducting a literature review of a child and adolescent forensic topic and with a written product suitable for publication submission
2. Writing an analysis and commentary of a recent landmark legal case that focuses on a legal issue related to children and adolescents with submission for publication
3. Writing a grant proposal and/or an Institutional Review Board protocol for a proposed research activity
4. Collaborating with a faculty member with an ongoing child and adolescent–focused forensic psychiatry research project

5. Preparation of a scholarly review of a child-focused forensic topic to be presented in a grand rounds format at a local or national meeting.

SUMMARY

Child and adolescent forensic psychiatry is a growing subspecialty, but exposure to child and adolescent forensic issues is extremely limited in both general psychiatry residency and child and adolescent psychiatry residency programs. Currently, there is no ACGME-approved Graduate Medical Education Program for child and adolescent forensic psychiatry. However, forensic psychiatry residency directors can create a child-focused forensic training opportunity that simultaneously meets the needs of the ACGME program in forensic psychiatry. By carefully creating didactic, clinical, and research experiences relevant to child and adolescent forensic psychiatric issues, forensic psychiatry program directors can provide this much-needed training to qualified psychiatrists.

REFERENCES

1. ACGME Program Requirements for Graduate Medical Education in Psychiatry. Available at: http://www.acgme.org/acWebsite/downloads/RRC_progReq/400_psychiatry_07012007_u04122008.pdf. Accessed October 6, 2010.
2. ACGME Program Requirements for Graduate Medical Education in Child and Adolescent Psychiatry. Available at: http://www.acgme.org/acWebsite/downloads/RRC_progReq/405pr07012007.pdf. Accessed October 6, 2010.
3. ACGME Program Requirements for Graduate Medical Education in Forensic Psychiatry. Available at: http://www.acgme.org/acwebsite/downloads/rrc_progreq/406pr703_u105.pdf. Accessed October 6, 2010.

An Annotated Bibliography for the Testifying Child and Adolescent Psychiatrist

Peter Ash, MD[a],*, Paul J. O'Leary, MD[b]

KEYWORDS

- Bibliography • Research • Juvenile • Child psychiatry
- Psychiatry • Forensic psychiatry

Dr Andrew Watson, a pioneer in child and adolescent forensic psychiatry, when trying to reduce residents' anxiety about undergoing cross-examination, was fond of saying, somewhat tongue-in-cheek, "There's nothing easier to testify about than your opinion." He was pointing out that experts can assert their opinions with or without a solid basis for them. Inherent in the concept of a hired gun is the idea that an expert can provide an opinion without a sound foundation.

However, convincing a judge or jury that an opinion is correct usually requires providing a sound basis for the opinion. Much of that basis involves laying out the relevant facts, and then explaining a clear reasoning process that moves from those facts to a conclusion. Often, it is useful to cite professional literature to back up the opinions or defend one's procedures. In jurisdictions that function under Daubert rules for the admissibility of expert testimony, there may be a challenge to the scientific basis for an expert opinion in a so-called Daubert hearing before trial. At such hearings, citing literature is almost always required to support the claim that the expert's opinion relies on scientific facts or proceeds from scientific methodology.

This annotated bibliography provides a sampling of articles that may be useful in supporting testimony. There is an extensive literature relevant to forensic child and adolescent psychiatry, and the small sample selected here is not comprehensive.

The authors have nothing to disclose.
[a] Psychiatry and Law Service, Division of Child and Adolescent Psychiatry, Department of Psychiatry and Behavioral Sciences, Emory University, Atlanta, GA, USA
[b] Psychiatry and Law Service, Department of Psychiatry and Behavioral Sciences, Emory University, Atlanta, GA, USA
* Corresponding author. Child Psychiatry, Suite 312-S, 1256 Briarcliff Road Northeast, Atlanta, GA 30306.
E-mail address: peter.ash@emory.edu

Child Adolesc Psychiatric Clin N Am 20 (2011) 577–590
doi:10.1016/j.chc.2011.03.001
1056-4993/11/$ – see front matter © 2011 Elsevier Inc. All rights reserved.

The publications selected here are examples of literature that may be cited by experts. Several criteria were used in selecting publications, including:

- Frequency with which the issue addressed arises in litigation
- How recently the reference was published
- Degree to which the reference includes a good summary of previous research
- Authority of the source, including whether the work was peer-reviewed
- Availability of full text online.

Beyond that, the selections reflect the attitudes, experience, judgments, and biases of the authors. Others would no doubt come up with different choices. It is the authors' hope that reading our selections will spur practitioners to come up with their own lists of useful references.

On a cautionary note, it should be emphasized that this bibliography is only a pointer to selected articles in the literature. Before referencing an article in a forensic report, in deposition, or in court testimony, the forensic expert should obtain a copy of the full article and read it carefully. Citing articles if one has only read the abstract leaves a witness vulnerable on cross-examination to unpleasant and embarrassing surprises if an attorney is able to point out that the article also contains data or statements that do not support the expert's position.

GENERAL TEXTBOOKS

Benedek EP, Ash P, Scott CL, editors. Principles and practice of child and adolescent forensic mental health. Washington, DC: American Psychiatric Publishing; 2010.

This recently revised textbook has 33 chapters that cover a wide variety of topics in child and adolescent forensic psychiatry. Each chapter has numerous references that direct the reader to research in the area covered. The book is an updating and expansion of the previous text *Principles and Practice of Child and Adolescent Forensic Psychiatry*. It can be cited as a standard reference in the field.

Sparta SN, Koocher GP, editors. Forensic mental health assessment of children and adolescents. New York: Oxford University Press; 2006.

This issue is a second general work edited and largely written by psychologists. It also provides discussion of a wide variety of child and adolescent forensic evaluations.

ABUSE AND NEGLECT: ASSESSMENT

American Academy of Child & Adolescent Psychiatry. Practice parameters for the forensic evaluation of children and adolescents who may have been physically or sexually abused. J Am Acad Child Adolesc Psychiatry 1997;36:423–42.

This document was developed by a group of forensic experts and it was approved by the Council of the American Academy of Child and Adolescent Psychiatry (AACAP). Practice parameters are generally written to encompass a wide variety of approaches. This parameter provides a standard that forensic psychiatrists can use to defend their examination procedures. Conversely, experts who do not abide by the practice parameter need to be prepared to defend their deviation from those practices.

Anderst J, Kellogg N, Jung I. Reports of repetitive penile-genital penetration often have no definitive evidence of penetration. Pediatrics 2009;124:403–9.

Whether negative results on physical examination indicate that no penile penetration occurred is a question that frequently arises in sexual abuse cases. This large-scale, recent study documents that a lack of physical findings is common in children who have been sexually abused.

Friedrich WN, Fisher JL, Dittner CA, et al. Child Sexual Behavior Inventory: normative, psychiatric, and sexual abuse comparisons. Child Maltreat 2001; 6:37–49.

The issue of whether unusual sexual behaviors are consequences of sexual abuse arises in a variety of cases. In evaluating children who may have been sexually abused, it is important to distinguish normal or typical sexual behaviors from abuse-related sexual behaviors. The Child Sexual Behavior Inventory has been widely accepted for that purpose. However, the research also points out that such behaviors are also more common in nonabused psychiatric outpatients than in normal children.

Malloy LC, Lyon TD, Quas JA. Filial dependency and recantation of child sexual abuse allegations. J Am Acad Child Adolesc Psychiatry 2007;46:162–70.

When a child recants a previous allegation of sexual abuse, how should this be understood? In this study, about one-quarter of children recanted at some point in the process. The investigators' data suggest that children recanted most commonly as a result of parental pressure, rather than out of a wish to correct a previous false allegation.

Orbach Y, Hershkowitz I, Lamb ME, et al. Assessing the value of structured protocols for forensic interviews of alleged child abuse victims. Child Abuse Negl 2000;24:733–52.

In sex abuse evaluations, how useful or misleading is it to ask specific, focused questions? In the face of earlier research showing that even experienced forensic investigators used many leading questions when interviewing children, this study examined the effects of using a scripted protocol developed by the National Institute of Child Health and Human Development (NICHD). The findings suggested that more details were obtained using open-ended questions. The article includes the NICHD protocol in an appendix.

Watkeys JM, Price LD, Upton PM, et al. The timing of medical examination following an allegation of sexual abuse: is this an emergency? Arch Dis Child 2008; 93:851–6.

Evaluators in sexual abuse cases may need to integrate the presence or absence of physical findings into their conclusions. This study presents recent data regarding the likelihood of physical findings and the effect of the timing of the examination. Of the girls in this study who were seen after an allegation of abuse, about half had physical findings when examined within a week of the alleged abuse, but the likelihood of physical findings was significantly lower when the examination occurred more than a week after the alleged abuse.

ABUSE AND NEGLECT: EFFECTS OF TESTIFYING ON CHILDREN

Goodman GS, Taub EP, Jones DP, et al. Testifying in criminal court: emotional effects on child sexual assault victims. Monogr Soc Res Child Dev 1992;57:1–142.

Many participants in trials involving sexual abuse are concerned about the possible detrimental effects on children from testifying. This study brings some data to bear on the question of how much psychological risk there is to the child, which variables affect that risk, and what steps to prepare the child might reduce the risk.

ABUSE AND NEGLECT: FOSTER CARE

Kessler RC, Pecora PJ, Williams J, et al. Effects of enhanced foster care on the long-term physical and mental health of foster care alumni. Arch Gen Psychiatry 2008;65:625–33.

Although child abuse and neglect are important risk factors for adult mental disorders, there are limited data on the effectiveness of treatment in the foster care system in ameliorating this risk. This study compared the outcomes of children in 2 public foster systems with the outcomes of children placed in a private, model foster care program that provided more services, and found that, overall, youth who received more intensive services did better.

Rubin DM, O'Reilly AL, Luan X, et al. The impact of placement stability on behavioral well-being for children in foster care. Pediatrics 2007;119:336–44.

Children in foster care frequently undergo change of placement, which is generally believed to be disruptive to children. However, the causal link between number of placements and outcomes is complicated by children with multiple placements often being moved because of disruptive behavior. This study provides data supporting the argument that multiple placements place children at risk independently of their baseline disruptive behaviors.

ABUSE AND NEGLECT: OUTCOMES

Scott KM, Smith DR, Ellis PM. Prospectively ascertained child maltreatment and its association with DSM-IV mental disorders in young adults. Arch Gen Psychiatry 2010;67:712–9.

What are the expected outcomes of child abuse? The research in this area has expanded, and the methodologies have improved. Although most studies use a retrospective design, this recent study from New Zealand uses a prospective ascertainment of abuse. The results suggest that abused children were at the highest risk for posttraumatic stress disorder (PTSD) and were at increased risk for mood, anxiety, and substance use disorders.

Bernet W, Corwin D. An evidence-based approach for estimating present and future damages from child sexual abuse. J Am Acad Psychiatry Law 2006; 34:224–30.

Estimating prognosis and future damages is a matter of integrating case specifics with research. This article addresses how to use relevant research in estimating damages in sexual abuse cases.

ABUSE AND NEGLECT: SUGGESTIBILITY

Ceci SJ, Kulkofsky S, Klemfuss JZ, et al. Unwarranted assumptions about children's testimonial accuracy. Annu Rev Clin Psychol 2007;3:311–28.

Whether a child's allegation of sexual abuse is accurate or the result of suggestion is a frequent issue in child sex abuse cases. Ceci and colleagues have reviewed their (and others') work in numerous publications. This publication is one of the more recent ones, and gives references back to the original data.

Ceci SJ, Bruck, M. Jeopardy in the courtroom: a scientific analysis of children's testimony. Washington, DC: American Psychological Association; 1995.

This book is a classic on the forensic implications of suggestibility in interviewing children. Although there has continued to be considerable research in this area since the book's publication, the detailed discussion and numerous examples possible in a book format make it still well worth reading.

ADOPTION

Keyes MA, Sharma A, Elkins IJ, et al. The mental health of US adolescents adopted in infancy. Arch Pediatr Adolesc Med 2008;162:419–25.

The question of whether adopted children are at risk for mental disorders has been the focus of a moderate amount of research. In this study comparing groups of adolescents, although most adopted adolescents were doing well, adoptees had moderately higher rates of mental health problems. Domestic adoptees were more likely to have an externalizing disorder than international adoptees.

Mallon GP. Assessing lesbian and gay prospective foster and adoptive families: a focus on the home study process. Child Welfare 2007;86:67–86.

Gay parent adoption is a growing, but still controversial, phenomenon. The general finding in the literature is that children of gay parents have been found to do as well as children of heterosexual parents. However, applying such group findings in an individual case is problematic. This article discusses specific factors to address in assessing gay parents as prospective parents.

DELINQUENCY

Snyder HN, Sickmund M. Juvenile offenders and victims: 2006 national report. Washington, DC: Office of Juvenile Justice and Delinquency Prevention; 2006.

The US Office of Juvenile Justice and Delinquency Prevention (OJJDP) is an excellent resource for statistics and publications related to delinquency. Most of their material is available online. See their Web site at http://www.ojjdp.gov/publications. The 2006 National Report collates data from US Federal Bureau of Investigation reports, surveys of juvenile detention facilities, and other sources to provide a view of juvenile crime and the justice system's response.

U.S. Department of Health and Human Services. Youth violence: a report of the surgeon general. Rockville (MD): US Department of Health and Human Services; 2001.

The Surgeon General's Report is an excellent synthesis of theories and statistics related to delinquency and its course. Among other issues, it discusses the high frequency of violence among adolescents (30%–40% of boys have committed a serious violent offense) and documents that only a small proportion of violent juvenile offenders go on to become adult criminals. The status of its author gives it a level of credibility that few scientific articles achieve.

DELINQUENCY: COMPETENCY TO STAND TRIAL

Grisso T, Steinberg L, Woolard J, et al. Juveniles' competence to stand trial: a comparison of adolescents' and adults' capacities as trial defendants. Law Hum Behav 2003;27:333–63.

Although competency to stand trial is an individualized assessment, evaluators are often asked to address how unusual it is for an adolescent of a particular age to be competent based on age and other developmental considerations. This study, using the MacArthur Competence Assessment Tool - Criminal Adjudication (MCAT-CA) and a measure of judgment, provides normative data to help answer those questions.

Mossman D, Noffsinger SG, Ash P, et al. AAPL practice guideline for the forensic psychiatric evaluation of competence to stand trial. J Am Acad Psychiatry Law 2007;35:S3–72.

This practice guideline developed by the American Academy of Psychiatry and the Law (AAPL) provides guidance and standards for conducting an evaluation for competence to stand trial (CST). The guideline includes a section discussing special issues that arise in the evaluation of juveniles. In addition, the guideline provides an extensive literature review and a table summarizing state statutes on CST.

DELINQUENCY: EXPOSURE TO MEDIA VIOLENCE

Anderson CA, Shibuya A, Ihori N, et al. Violent video game effects on aggression, empathy, and prosocial behavior in eastern and western countries: a meta-analytic review. Psychol Bull 2010;136:151–73.

Whether youth should be allowed to buy and use violent video games is a controversial public policy question. This meta-analysis suggests that playing violent video games is a causal risk factor for increased aggressive behavior, aggressive cognition, and aggressive affect. The paper contains an extensive bibliography of research in the area.

Council on Communications and Media. American Academy of Pediatrics: policy statement: media violence. Pediatrics 2009;124:1495–503.

The American Academy of Pediatrics has taken the position that violence in media represents a significant risk to the health of children and adolescents. This position paper summarizes their view of the research and provides references.

Ybarra ML, Diener-West M, Markow D, et al. Linkages between internet and other media violence with seriously violent behavior by youth. Pediatrics 2008; 122:929–37.

The existence of a causal link between adolescent exposure to violence in media and committing violent acts is controversial. This large-scale study finds an association between exposure through media and action, but leaves open whether there is a causal link.

DELINQUENCY: JUVENILE CULPABILITY

Cauffman E, Steinberg L. (Im)maturity of judgment in adolescence: why adolescents may be less culpable than adults. Behav Sci Law 2000;18:741–60.

This classic article provides a research basis for saying that immaturity of judgment in adolescents is grounds for holding adolescents less criminally responsible even when their logical reasoning is similar to that of adults.

Giedd JN. The teen brain: insights from neuroimaging. J Adolesc Health 2008;42: 335–43.

Immaturity of the adolescent brain is now often cited as supporting the proposition that there is a biologic structural basis for poor judgment in the developing adolescent brain, and that this poor judgment should be a mitigating factor when an adolescent commits a crime. This paper summarizes results of the National Institute of Mental Health (NIMH) longitudinal study of brain development and reports on data from 2000 subjects. The paper discusses specific brain regions, how their interconnectedness increases with development, how their morphology changes with development, and how these changes affect behavior. Particular attention is paid to how the development and integration of executive functioning and the reward and motivational systems affect adolescent behavior.

Steinberg L, Scott ES. Less guilty by reason of adolescence: developmental immaturity, diminished responsibility, and the juvenile death penalty. Am Psychol 2003;58:1009–18.

The US Supreme Court decision Roper v Simmons, which ended the death penalty for juveniles, cited this article multiple times and largely adopted the reasoning outlined in this paper: that adolescents are less culpable because (1) their decision-making capacity is not mature, (2) they are subject to adverse environmental coercion that they cannot escape, and (3) their characters are still undergoing change. These categories have persisted in arguments for mitigated sentencing of juvenile and were reiterated in the 2009 Supreme Court decisions eliminating life without parole sentences for juveniles for crimes less than murder. These concepts have clear applicability in cases dealing with mitigation of responsibility for juvenile offenders and should be taken into account in sentencing.

DELINQUENCY: PSYCHOPATHY

Edens JF, Campbell JS, Weir JM. Youth psychopathy and criminal recidivism: a meta-analysis of the psychopathy checklist measures. Law Hum Behav 2007; 31:53–75.

The construct of psychopathy in adolescence has received considerable attention, in large part because of questions about what the diagnosis portends in terms of future course. This review suggests that youth psychopathy is statistically, although weakly, associated with general and violent recidivism, but negligibly related to sexual recidivism.

Lynam DR, Caspi A, Moffitt TE, et al. Longitudinal evidence that psychopathy scores in early adolescence predict adult psychopathy. J Abnorm Psychol 2007; 116:155–65.

Psychopathy in adolescence has received considerable recent attention, in large part because, in adults, psychopathy is strongly associated with recidivism and resistance to treatment. In the juvenile literature, the picture is less clear, and one of the major questions is the degree to which psychopathy diagnosed in adolescence persists into adulthood. This study assessed adolescents at age 13 years and again at age 24 years. Although there were significant associations such that the investigators conclude that psychopathy is moderately stable, they also note that the positive predictive power (the likelihood that a boy diagnosed with psychopathy at age 13 years will later meet criteria at age 24 years) is poor, a finding in line with previous work suggesting that a finding of psychopathy in adolescence has limited value in making predictions in an individual case.

DELINQUENCY: RISK ASSESSMENT

Borum R, Verhaagen D. Assessing and managing violence risk in juveniles. New York: Guilford Press; 2006.

This book is a comprehensive resource on issues involved in risk assessment in youth. It provides a good review of research in the area of juvenile risk assessment as well as integrating the research into formulating risk assessment reports.

Catchpole REH, Gretton HM. The predictive validity of risk assessment with violent young offenders. A 1-year examination of criminal outcome. Crim Justice Behav 2003;30:688–708.

For juveniles, the risk of reoffending is often important in sentencing determinations. This study assesses the predictive accuracy of 3 standard instruments (the Structured Assessment of Violence Risk in Youth, the Youth Level of Service/Case Management Inventory, and the Psychopathy Checklist: Youth Version) and finds a moderate to strong relationship between each and reoffending within 1 year.

DELINQUENCY: SEXUAL OFFENDERS

Seto MC, Lalumiere ML. What is so special about male adolescent sexual offending? A review and test of explanations through meta-analysis. Psychol Bull 2010;136:526–75.

This is a long paper that discusses several theories of sexual offending in the context of a meta-analysis of 59 studies that compared male adolescent sex offenders with other male adolescent offenders. Although there were many similarities between adolescent sex and non–sex offenders, the study concluded that the general delinquency explanation is not sufficient to understand adolescent sexual offending. The largest group difference was attributable to atypical sexual interests, followed by sexual abuse history, criminal history, antisocial associations, and substance abuse.

Worling JR, Litteljohn A, Bookalam D. 20-year prospective follow-up study of specialized treatment for adolescents who offended sexually. Behav Sci Law 2010;28:46–57.

A common question in the sentencing of adolescent sexual offenders is the degree to which a rehabilitative approach is likely to be successful. Adolescents are often seen by judges as more amenable to treatment than adults. This prospective study of the treatment effectiveness of a Canadian sample found that treatment reduced recidivism to about half the rate of the nontreated comparison group across all domains of offending: sexual, violent, and nonviolent. The 20-year recidivism rate of the treated sexual offenders was less than 10%.

DIVORCE AND CHILD CUSTODY

American Academy of Child and Adolescent Psychiatry. Practice parameters for child custody evaluation. J Am Acad Child Adolesc Psychiatry 1997;36:57S–68S.

This practice parameter was developed by a group of forensic experts and then approved by the Council of the AACAP. Practice parameters are generally written to encompass a wide variety of approaches. This parameter provides a standard that forensic experts can use to defend their evaluation procedures. Conversely, experts who do not abide by the practice parameter need to be prepared to defend their deviation from those practices.

Ash P, Guyer MJ. Biased reporting by parents undergoing child custody evaluations. J Am Acad Child Adolesc Psychiatry 1991;30:835–8.

Forensic evaluators often think that parents are distorting their reports of their children's functioning in a direction that supports the parents' position in litigation. However, without clear evidence of lying, an evaluator may have difficulty supporting such a judgment under cross-examination. This article provides a research basis for suspecting that distortion is common.

Bernet W, editor. Parental alienation, DSM-5, and ICD-11. Springfield (IL): Charles C Thomas; 2010.

This book outlines the research that supports the validity of parental alienation as a concept, the reliability of the diagnostic criteria, and the estimated prevalence of this condition. The bibliography of this book contains more than 500 references regarding parental alienation from 30 countries and supports the premise that the concept of parental alienation is generally accepted by the professional community.

Galatzer-Levy RM, Kraus L, Galatzer-Levy J, editors. The scientific basis of child custody decisions. 2nd edition. Hoboken (NJ): John Wiley; 2009.

The question of how much science there is in making child custody recommendations in divorce is contested. The chapters of this book provide extensive discussion of the research basis for different aspects of custody recommendations. Each chapter includes extensive references to the relevant research studies.

Johnston JR, Kline M, Tschann JM. Ongoing postdivorce conflict: effects on children of joint custody and frequent access. Am J Orthopsychiatry 1989;59:576–92.

The question of when joint custody should be recommended when parents contest custody frequently arises in custody evaluations. This study and others it cites suggest that, for couples who have a high level of conflict, joint custody may be disadvantageous to children.

Tippins TM, Wittmann JP. Empirical and ethical problems with custody recommendations: a call for clinical humility and judicial vigilance. Fam Court Rev 2005;43:193–222.

Research findings apply to sample groups, and the issue of how to apply research findings to an individual case is complex. In this article, the investigators argue that, because of the state of research on custody outcomes and the nature of making recommendations in a judicial setting, custody evaluators should not make specific recommendations about custody to the courts.

DIVORCE AND CHILD CUSTODY: SAME-SEX PARENTS

Rosenfeld MJ. Nontraditional families and childhood progress through school. Demography 2010;47:755–75.

How children fare when being raised by gay parents is an issue in some custody cases as well as in the public debate about gay marriage. The mental health literature has generally shown that children do as well when raised by 2 gay parents as by heterosexual parents, but that research has been criticized for having small samples. This study uses US census data to overcome that criticism, but does have the limitation of using school retention as a proxy for problems in development. The results show that children of same-sex couples are as likely to make normal progress through school as the children of most other family structures. The paper also provides a good review of the mental health research in the field.

Wainright JL, Russell ST, Patterson CJ. Psychosocial adjustment, school outcomes, and romantic relationships of adolescents with same-sex parents. Child Dev 2004;75:1886–98.

Studies of children of gay parents have not found consistent differences in their adjustment compared with the adjustment of children raised by heterosexual parents. This study draws its samples from a national sample of adolescents, and so overcomes some of the sampling problems found in earlier research. The investigators found that adolescents were functioning well, and that their adjustment was not generally associated with family type.

ETHICS

American Academy of Child & Adolescent Psychiatry (2009). Code of ethics. Available at: http://www.aacap.org/galleries/AboutUs/AACAP_Code_of_Ethics. pdf. Accessed November 26, 2010.

The AACAP is a national organization of physicians who treat children with regard to mental health. The ethical guidelines serve as a framework for practitioners in child and adolescent mental health with regard to their interactions with patients and their families. The document also details that AACAP subscribes to the Principles of Medical Ethics of the American Medical Association (AMA), in particular the Annotations Especially Applicable to Psychiatry.

American Academy of Psychiatry and the Law (2005). Ethics guidelines for the practice of forensic psychiatry. Available at: http://www.aapl.org/ethics.htm. Accessed February 4, 2011.

The American Academy of Psychiatry and the Law (AAPL) is the leading organization of forensic psychiatrists. Although the AAPL ethics guidelines technically apply only to members of AAPL, they nevertheless provide standards for the conduct of forensic evaluations. Evaluators who deviate from these standards can expect to be cross-examined on their deviations.

American Medical Association (2010). Code of medical ethics of the American Medical Association. Available at: http://www.ama-assn.org/ama/pub/physician-resources/medical-ethics/code-medical-ethics.shtml. Accessed November 26, 2010.

In 1847, the AMA established uniform standards for its members' professional education, training, and conduct. The Code of Medical Ethics has been updated several times, and the current version consists of 9 principles. For instance, the first principle is, "A physician shall be dedicated to providing competent medical care, with compassion and respect for human dignity and rights." The AMA also publishes opinions on ethical topics that relate the basic principles to actual practice.

MALPRACTICE AND REGULATION OF PRACTICE: PRESCRIBING

Bazzano ATF, Mangione-Smith R, Schonlau M, et al. Off-label prescribing to children in the United States outpatient setting. Acad Pediatr 2009;9:81–8.

In many child and adolescent psychiatry cases involving medication, psychiatrists are criticized for the off-label use of medication. This study, although not specific to psychiatry, documents that off-label prescribing is common, occurring in about two-thirds of outpatient visits.

Hammad TA, Laughren T, Racoosin J. Suicidality in pediatric patients treated with antidepressant drugs. Arch Gen Psychiatry 2006;63:332–9.

The black-box warning mandated by the US Food and Drug Administration (FDA) for selective serotonin reuptake inhibitors (SSRIs) for adolescents has been controversial, especially among child and adolescent psychiatrists. This was one of the early and influential analyses of drug trial data that showed a modest increase in risk of reported suicidality.

Morrato EH, Libby AM, Orton HD, et al. Frequency of provider contact after FDA advisory on risk of pediatric suicidality with SSRIs. Am J Psychiatry 2008;165: 42–50.

The FDA black-box warning for SSRIs for youth included a recommendation of weekly monitoring for suicidality when an SSRI is first started. The results of this study suggest that clinicians have not significantly increased their monitoring in response, which arguably bears on the question of what is the standard of practice.

Shah SS, Hall M, Goodman DM, et al. Off-label drug use in hospitalized children. Arch Pediatr Adolesc Med 2007;161:282–90.

In many child and adolescent psychiatry cases involving medication, psychiatrists are criticized for the off-label use of medication. This large-scale study, although not specific to psychiatry, documents that off-label prescribing is common in inpatient settings, occurring in more than three-quarters of cases.

MALPRACTICE AND REGULATION OF PRACTICE: SUICIDE

American Academy of Child and Adolescent Psychiatry. Practice parameter for the assessment and treatment of children and adolescents with suicidal behavior. J Am Acad Child Adolesc Psychiatry 2001;40:24S–51S.

This practice parameter developed by the AACAP provides guidelines and identifies minimal standards for the assessment of suicidality in adolescents. In addition, it summarizes the evidence for the effectiveness of a range of interventions. It also provides a balanced literature review and lists of resources.

Brent DA, Baugher M, Birmaher B, et al. Compliance with recommendations to remove firearms in families participating in a clinical trial for adolescent depression. J Am Acad Child Adolesc Psychiatry 2000;39:1220–6.

In a malpractice case involving an adolescent committing suicide with a gun, a question often arises as to whether the clinician recommended that the family remove guns from the home. If the defendant doctor failed to make such a recommendation, and this is held to be less than the standard of practice, the plaintiff must still prove that such a failure is the proximate cause of the suicide. This study documents the low level of compliance with such a recommendation.

Grunbaum JA, Kann L, Kinchen S, et al. Youth risk behavior surveillance – United States, 2003. MMWR Surveill Summ 2004;53:1–96.

In malpractice cases stemming from an outpatient youth suicide, the ability to foresee suicide is often a central question. This government report documents high rates of youth risk-taking behaviors. It documents that about 1 in 12 adolescents have made a suicide attempt in the preceding year, which implies that, even among that group, completed suicide is a rare event.

Marttunen MJ, Aro HM, Lonnqvist JK. Precipitant stressors in adolescent suicide. J Am Acad Child Adolesc Psychiatry 1993;32:1178–83.

In a malpractice case arising from an adolescent suicide, there are often questions about whether the suicide was a consequence of an inadequate risk assessment by the clinician, whether the suicide was reasonably foreseeable, and whether there was some intervening cause after the last therapy appointment that caused the tragic result. This study found that, in a Finnish sample of adolescents, more than two-thirds of completed suicides had a clear precipitant. In about half the cases, the precipitant occurred in the 24 hours preceding the suicide.

PERSONAL INJURY

Ackerman JP, Riggins T, Black MM. A review of the effects of prenatal cocaine exposure among school-aged children. Pediatrics 2010;125:554–65.

The crack baby issue arises in a variety of legal cases, including prosecutions of the mother for delivering cocaine to the fetus. Most research has found that prenatal cocaine exposure (PCE) has no demonstrable effects on preschool children. This paper reviews the research on school-aged children and suggests that the associations between PCE and growth, cognitive ability, academic achievement, and language functioning were difficult to distinguish from environmental variables. However, in school-age children, when environmental variables were statistically controlled, PCE did have a small but significant negative association with sustained attention and behavioral self-regulation.

Copeland WE, Keeler G, Angold A, et al. Traumatic events and posttraumatic stress in childhood. Arch Gen Psychiatry 2007;64:577–84.

Although many studies of trauma emphasize the frequency of later psychological disorders, this study found that few who experienced trauma developed full PTSD. Of children aged 9 to 13 years who were studied annually until they were 16 years old, more than two-thirds of the children reported at least 1 trauma. Many developed some symptoms, but, for many, effects were brief and even fewer met full criteria for PTSD. The study also identified variables that predicted higher rates of PTSD for certain subgroups.

Holbrook TL, Hoyt DB, Coimbra R, et al. High rates of acute stress disorder impact quality-of-life outcomes in injured adolescents: mechanism and gender predict acute stress disorder risk. J Trauma 2005;59:1126–30.

What is the evidence base for predicting long-term psychiatric damage from physical trauma? This study of 401 adolescent trauma patients found that acute stress disorder was strongly associated with significant reductions in quality of life measured at 2-year follow-up.

National Center for Injury Prevention and Control (2010). Injury prevention & control: data & statistics (WISQARS). Available at: http://www.cdc.gov/injury/wisqars/index.html. Accessed September 28, 2010.

It is often helpful to have reliable data about causes of injury and death. Web-based Injury Statistics Query and Reporting System (WISQARS) is an interactive database system maintained by the Centers for Disease Control and Prevention (CDC) that provides customized reports of injury-related data.

Storr CL, Ialongo NS, Anthony JC, et al. Childhood antecedents of exposure to traumatic events and posttraumatic stress disorder. Am J Psychiatry 2007; 164:119–25.

Not all children who are exposed to trauma develop PTSD, and a good deal of research is being done to identify the factors that discriminate which children exposed to trauma are at highest risk. In this large-sample, prospective study, first-graders with high self-rated depressive and anxious symptoms were found to be moderately more at risk when reassessed as young adults. Young adults who scored in the highest quartile on a reading test in the first grade were at lower risk for exposure to assaultive violence traumas.

SCHOOL

Sattler JM. Assessment of children: cognitive foundations. 5th edition. San Diego (CA): J.M. Sattler; 2008.

Evaluations for special education services typically include cognitive assessment. This volume is a standard reference on the use of cognitive assessments of children. It is not a manual that teaches how to administer tests, but rather guides the interpretation of test results. Although the book emphasizes the interpretation of the Wechsler intelligence quotient (IQ) tests, it also addresses more specialized IQ and development measures sometimes seen in school assessments.

US Department of Education (2010). Q and A: questions and answers on individualized education programs (IEP's), evaluations and reevaluations. Available at: http://idea.ed.gov/explore/view/p/%2Croot%2Cdynamic%2CQaCorner%2C3%2C. Accessed October 29, 2010.

The individualized educational program (IEP) is the cornerstone of the process of providing special education services. Such services are provided under federal law, and the rules governing the processes are complex. Forensic reports regarding educational services are an exception to the general rule of writing in layman's language; in these reports, the jargon needs to be used in accordance with legal defi-nitions. This question and answer prepared by the US Department of Education is a useful guide to those who are involved in litigation involving special education services.

SCHOOL: BULLYING

Arseneault L, Walsh E, Trzesniewski K, et al. Bullying victimization uniquely contributes to adjustment problems in young children: a nationally representative cohort study. Pediatrics 2006;118:130–8.

With greater understanding of bullying at school, cases involving allegations of a school's failure to respond to bullying have been increasing. This large-scale study provides data on potential damage suffered from bullying.

Sourander A, Brunstein Klomek A, Ikonen M, et al. Psychosocial risk factors associated with cyberbullying among adolescents: a population-based study. Arch Gen Psychiatry 2010;67:720–8.

Cyberbullying is becoming a new area for research. This large-scale study of Finnish adolescents examined psychosocial and psychiatric risk factors associated with cyberbullying. Both being the cyberbully and being the victim were found to be associated with mental health and psychosomatic problems.

ACKNOWLEDGMENTS

The authors thank William Bernet, MD, Fabian M. Saleh, MD, and Philip Stahl, PhD, for suggesting references to include in this bibliography.

Index

Note: Page numbers of article titles are in **boldface** type.

A

Abuse and neglect, annotated bibliography for testifying child and adolescent psychiatrist related to
  assessment-related information, 578–579
  effects of testifying on children, 579–580
  foster care–related, 580
  outcomes-related, 580
  suggestibility, 580–581
Accidental indoctrination, contact refusal by children of divorce related to, 472–473
ACGME. See *American Council on Graduate Medical Education (ACGME).*
Achenbach Child Behavior Checklist (CBCL), 550
Adolescent Psychopathology Scale, 551
Adoption, annotated bibliography for testifying child and adolescent psychiatrist related to, 581
Aggressor(s), in bullying, functional assessment of, 453, 455–456, 458
American Council on Graduate Medical Education (ACGME), 565
  child-focused learning sites of, 568–569
  child-focused track of, specialty curriculum for, 569–572
  forensic experiences, 572–574
  forensic psychiatry teaching faculty of, 567–568
  forensic requirements of, 566–567
  resident scholarly activity in, 574
Annotated bibliography, for testifying child and adolescent psychiatrist, **577–590.** See also specific subject matter and *Child and adolescent psychiatrist, testifying, annotated bibliography.*

B

Behavior Assessment System for Children-2 (BASC-2), 550–551
Behavioral problems, child maltreatment and, 506
Brain
  abnormalities of, forensic neuroimaging for, 540
  images of, normalization of, forensic neuroimaging in, 541
Bullying
  aggressors in, functional assessment of, 453, 455–456, 458
  annotated bibliography for testifying child and adolescent psychiatrist related to, 590
  approach to, **447–465**
    conceptual, 450–454
    tactics to get out of corners, 460–463
      for cyberbullying, 462–463
      in elementary school, 460–461
      in high school, 462

Child Adolesc Psychiatric Clin N Am 20 (2011) 591–599
doi:10.1016/S1056-4993(11)00052-6
1056-4993/11/$ – see front matter © 2011 Elsevier Inc. All rights reserved.

childpsych.theclinics.com

Moving?

Make sure your subscription moves with you!

To notify us of your new address, find your **Clinics Account Number** (located on your mailing label above your name), and contact customer service at:

Email: journalscustomerservice-usa@elsevier.com

800-654-2452 (subscribers in the U.S. & Canada)
314-447-8871 (subscribers outside of the U.S. & Canada)

Fax number: 314-447-8029

Elsevier Health Sciences Division
Subscription Customer Service
3251 Riverport Lane
Maryland Heights, MO 63043

*To ensure uninterrupted delivery of your subscription, please notify us at least 4 weeks in advance of move.